SELF-CARE

STAY YOUNGER AND LIVE LONGER

Professor M.S. Rao, Ph.D.
The Father of Soft Leadership

&

M. Padmavathy

Foreword By
Garry Ridge

STAGE PUBLISHING & PROMOTION CO.

Self-Care

Stay Younger And Live Longer

Professor M.S. Rao, Ph.D.
The Father of Soft Leadership

M. Padmavathy

Foreword By
Garry Ridge

Publisher:
Stage Publishing & Promotion Co.

Copyright Notice

Copyright © 2025 Stage Publishing & Promotion Co.
All Rights Reserved.

No part of this publication, including but not limited to Self-Care: Stay Younger and Live Longer, may be reproduced, stored in a database or retrieval system, or distributed, or transmitted in any form or by any means, including photocopying, recording, or other electronic or mechanical methods, without the prior written permission of the copyright holder, except in the case of brief quotations embodied in critical reviews and certain other noncommercial uses permitted by copyright law.

For permission requests, write to the copyright holder at the address below.

Stage PUBLISHING & Promotion Co.
PO Box 806 / Glendale, CA 91209-USA
ISBN: 978-1-966837-43-5

Printed in the United States of America

Table of Contents

Endorsements and Praises 9
Quotes 1
Preface 28
Authors' Note 30
Acknowledgments 31
1 – Practice Self-Care 33
2 – Describe Your Perfect Day 40
3 – Be the Best Version of Yourself 43
4 – Build Your Character to Become a Champion 47
5 – Improve Your Attitude 51
6 – Lead a Healthy Lifestyle 57
7 – Make Fitness an Integral Part of Your Life 61
8 – Participate in Physical Activities and Events 68
9 – Participate in Sports and Games Regularly 73
10 – Eat a Variety of Foods to Stay Healthy 76
11 – Boost Your Memory with the Right Foods 84
12 – Drink Water Adequately 90
13 – Overcome ADHD 95
14 – Detoxify Your Body, Mind, and Soul Periodically ... 100
15 – Be Image Conscious 104
16 – Pursue Modeling as a Career 109
17 – Explore Stoic Philosophy to Achieve Peace and Happiness 114
18 – Eat to Live, not Live to Eat 122
19 – Stay Younger and Live Longer 130
Epilogue 139
List of Books Published by the Author 141
Making a Positive Difference in the World 146
About The Book 147
About The Authors 149

Endorsements and Praises
for
Self-Care: Stay Younger and Live Longer

"Professor M.S. Rao and his wife M. Padmavathy explain how to lead a healthy lifestyle and build character to become a champion. They encourage participation in physical activities to make fitness an integral part of daily life. By outlining health, wealth, nutrition, fitness, and beauty, they increase purpose and meaning in your life. I wish I had this book long ago. I could have used it!"

Dave Ulrich
Rensis Likert Professor, Ross School of Business, University of Michigan - Partner, the RBL Group

"Professor M.S. Rao is recognized as the 'Father of Soft Leadership.' His latest work focuses on the need for leaders to protect their foundation of health, wealth, and family. Professor Rao's writing is compelling because he offers "lived words," based on his own extraordinary leadership journey."

James Strock,
Author, Serve to Lead

"*Self-Care* is a book for all leaders who want to pursue a healthy, balanced, and positive life! Leaders won't be happy and make a difference to others unless they are healthy psychologically, physically, and spiritually. I strongly endorse the views of *Self-Care* and recommend it to leaders anywhere—eat healthy, exercise regularly, live to make a difference, learn and share continuously, and love others!"

Arthur Yeung
President of YOLO, Adjunct Professor at China Europe International Business School

Quotes

"I slept and I dreamed that life is all joy. I woke and I saw that life is all service. I served and saw that service is a joy." Khalil Gibran

"Self-care is a divine responsibility." Danielle LaPorte

"Happiness is an attitude of the mind." Keshub Mahindra, Chairman Emeritus

"As you grow older, you will discover that you have two hands, one for helping yourself, the other for helping others." Maya Angelou

"There are two ways to live your life. One is to believe there are no miracles. Another to believe that everything is a miracle." Albert Einstein

"Youth is happy because it can see beauty. Anyone who keeps the ability to see beauty never grows old." Franz Kafka

"Nothing is impossible, the word itself says 'I'm possible'!" Audrey Hepburn

"To be the best in the world necessitates your drawing upon all your capacities. In the doing, you will draw on what is unique in yourself. No one can replicate it." James Strock

"He who lives in harmony with himself lives in harmony with the universe." Marcus Aurelius

"The root of all health is in the brain. The trunk of it is in emotion. The branches and leaves are the body. The flower of health blooms when all parts work together." Kurdish saying

"The progressive increase of data may cause the older brain to process all the information a bit more slowly, but we ultimately continue to become more intelligent with age." Christopher Bergland, *Psychology Today*

"The best bridge between despair and hope is a good night's sleep." E. Joseph Cossman

"Anyone who stops learning is old, whether at 20 or 80. Anyone who keeps learning stays young. The greatest thing in life is to keep your mind young!" Henry Ford

"It is better to wear out than to rust out!" Richard Cumberland

"Life is partly what we make it, and partly what it is made by the friends we choose." Tennessee Williams

"There is only one way to happiness and that is to cease worrying about things which are beyond the power of our will." Epictetus

"Pause, really sit back and imagine what your life would be like without that thing you take for granted." Alex Lickerman

"The best remedy for a short temper is a long walk." Anonymous

"A sad soul can kill you quicker than a germ." John Steinbeck

"True enjoyment comes from activity of the mind and exercise of the body; the two are ever united." Anonymous

"Pure water is the world's first and foremost medicine." Slovakian proverb

"Water is critical for sustainable development, including environmental integrity and the alleviation of poverty and hunger, and is indispensable for human health and well-being." United Nations

"Nothing would be more tiresome than eating and drinking if God had not made them a pleasure as well as a necessity." Voltaire

"The belly rules the mind." Spanish proverb

"You have power over your mind – not outside events. Realize this, and you will find strength." Marcus Aurelius

"Never bend your head. Always hold it high. Look the world straight in the face." Helen Keller

"The worst loneliness is not to be comfortable with yourself." Mark Twain

"The human body is the best picture of the human soul." Ludwig Wittgenstein

"Take care of your body. It's the only place you have to live." Jim Rohn

"The higher your energy level, the more efficient your body. The more efficient your body, the better you feel and the more you will use your talent to produce outstanding results." Anthony Robbins

"Health is the greatest of all possessions; a pale cobbler is better than a sick king." Isaac Bickerstaff

"If you're fifty, exercise your mind and body regularly, eat well, and have a general zest for life, you're likely younger – in very real, physical terms – than your neighbor who is forty-four, works in a dead-end job, eats chicken wings twice a day, considers thinking too strenuous, and looks at lifting a beer glass as a reasonable daily workout." Ken Robinson

"A man is born gentle and weak. At death, he is hard and stiff. Green plants are tender and filled with sap. At death, they are withered and dry. Therefore, the stiff and unbending is the disciple of death, and the gentle and yielding is the disciple of life." Lao Tzu

"The purpose of training is to tighten up the slack, toughen the body, and polish the spirit." Morihei Ueshiba

"There is no easy way out. If there were, I would have bought it. And believe me, it would be one of my favorite things." Oprah Winfrey

"Reading is to the mind what exercise is to the body." Joseph Addison

"I'm not in the best shape, but I want to prove to myself I can do something that seems insurmountable and inspire others by showing them no matter where they are in their fitness goals, they can do it, too." Ruben Studdard

"The mind is the most important part of achieving any fitness goal. Mental change always comes before physical change." Matt McGorry

"Exercise should be regarded as tribute to the heart." — Gene Tunney

"I don't smoke, don't drink much, and go to the gym five times a week. I live a healthy lifestyle and feel great. I can run a marathon, you know." Sarah Michelle Gellar

"A feeble body weakens the mind." Jean-Jacques Rousseau

"I've spent half my life in gyms, if not more, and I love physical fitness and health; couple that with the fact that I love for people to be healthy, whether it's mentally, physically, or emotionally, and it's just a great opportunity for me to do something I love and have an impact on people's health." Steve Nash

"Here's what I tell anybody and this is what I believe. The greatest gift we have is the gift of life. We understand that. That comes from our Creator. We're given a body. Now you may not like it, but you can maximize that body the best it can be maximized." Mike Ditka

"I think exercise tests us in so many ways, our skills, our hearts, our ability to bounce back after setbacks. This is the inner beauty of sports and competition, and it can serve us all well as adult athletes." Peggy Fleming

"Hardships often prepare ordinary people for an extraordinary destiny." C.S. Lewis

"Remember, to spend some time with your loved ones, because they are not going to be around forever. Remember to hold hands and cherish the moment for someday that person might not be there again. Give time to love, give time to speak! And give time to share the precious thoughts in your mind." Bob Moorehead

"We are different, in essence, from other men. If you want to win something, run 100 meters. If you want to EXPERIENCE something, run a marathon." Emil Zatopek, 1952 Olympic Marathon gold medalist

"Running is alone time that lets my brain unspool the tangles that build up over days…I run, pound it out on the pavement, channel that energy into my legs, and when I'm done with my run, I'm done with it." Rob Haneisen, runner

"Running allows me to set my mind free. Nothing seems impossible. Nothing unattainable." Kara Goucher, Olympic long-distance runner

"I think I get addicted to the feelings associated with the end of a long run. I love feeling empty, clean, worn out, and sweat-purged. I love that good ache of the muscles that have done me proud." Kristin Armstrong, *author of Mile Markers*

"It's very hard at the beginning to understand that the whole idea is not to beat the other runners. Eventually, you learn that the competition is against the little voice inside you that wants you to quit." George Sheehan, M.D., *author of Going the Distance*

"You have to wonder at times what you're doing out there. Over the years, I've given myself a thousand reasons to keep running, but it always comes back to where it started. It comes down to self-satisfaction and a sense of achievement." Steve Prefontaine, international track star

"The obsession with running is an obsession with the potential for more and more life." George Sheehan, M.D., author of Going the Distance

"Marathoning is like cutting yourself unexpectedly. You dip into the pain so gradually that the damage is done before you are aware of it. Unfortunately, when the awareness comes, it is excruciating." John Farrington

"The music of a marathon is a powerful strain, one of those tunes of glory. It asks us to forsake pleasures, to discipline the body, to find courage, to renew faith and to become one's person, utterly and completely." George Sheehan, *running author*

"If you want to become the best runner you can be, start now. Don't spend the rest of your life wondering if you could do it" Priscilla Welsh

"Confidence is not some nonphysical quality snatched from the spiritual dimension and installed in the mind. It is the feeling that arises when the body's knowledge of itself is in harmony with a person's dreams." Matt Fitzgerald

"Fitness has to be fun. If it isn't, there will be no fitness. Play is the process. Fitness is merely the product."

Dr. George Sheehan
"Noontime running provides a triple benefit: daylight, a break from the workday, and a chance to avoid eating a heavy lunch." Joe Henderson

"Visualizing perfect running form will help you stay relaxed. Visualize before the race. Then, once you're in the race, pick out someone who's looking good and running relaxed. This will help you do the same." Gayle Barron, *1978 Boston Marathon champion*

"Eat food. Not too much. Mostly plants." Michael Pollan

"Eating a high-nutrient diet makes you more satisfied with less food, and gives the ability to enjoy food more without overeating." Joel Fuhrman

"If you maintain a healthy diet, or at least are smart about your food choices, you'll still see the pounds come off." Misty May-Treanor

"Juices of fruits and vegetables are pure gifts from Mother Nature and the most natural way to heal your body and make yourself whole again." Farnoosh Brock

"Your mind is for having ideas, not holding them." David Allen

"Much of the stress that people feel doesn't come from having too much to do. It comes from not finishing what they've started." David Allen

"The greatest effect coming out of silence is the clarity one has in listening. Every note stands alone." Jack Dorsey, *CEO of Twitter*

"The more you sweat in peace, the less you bleed in war." Norman Schwarzkopf

"By the time you're eighty years old, you've learned everything. You only have to remember it." George Burns

"Aging is not lost youth but a new stage of opportunity and strength." Betty Friedan

"At age 20, we worry about what others think of us. At age 40, we don't care what they think of us. At age 60, we discover they haven't been thinking of us at all." Ann Landers

"A good youth ought to have a fear of God, to be subject to his parents, to give honor to his elders, to preserve his purity; he ought not to despise humility, but should love forbearance and modesty. All these are an ornament to youthful years." Saint Ambrose

"Youth is a blunder; Manhood a struggle, Old Age a regret." Benjamin Disraeli

"Most people say that it's the intellect which makes a great scientist. They are wrong: it is character." Albert Einstein

"Character isn't something you were born with and can't change, like your fingerprints. It's something you weren't born with and must take responsibility for forming." Jim Rohn

"Champions aren't made in gyms. Champions are made from something they have deep inside them desire, a dream, a vision. They have to have the skill and the will. But the will must be stronger than the skill." Muhammad Ali

"Losers live in the past. Winners learn from the past and enjoy working in the present toward the future." Denis Waitley

"Character is the result of two things: Mental attitude and the way we spend our time." Elbert Green Hubbard

"To be a champion, I think you have to see the big picture. It's not about winning and losing; it's about everyday hard work and about thriving on a challenge. It's about embracing the pain that you'll experience at the end of a race and not being afraid. I think people think too hard and get afraid of a certain challenge." Summer Sanders

"Men of character are the conscience of the society to which they belong." Ralph Waldo Emerson

"The greatest way to live with honor in this world is to be what we pretend to be." Socrates

"Of all the properties which belong to honorable men, not one is so highly prized as that of character." Henry Clay

"Put a rogue in the limelight and he will act like an honest man." Napoleon

"In the future, the learners will inherit the earth, while the learned will find themselves beautifully equipped to live in a world that no longer exists." Eric Hoffer, Philosopher

"Every single day is a good day no matter how bright or dark it is because it always brings an opportunity to start a positive beginning in your life." Edmond Mbiaka

"Having a positive mental attitude is asking how something can be done rather than saying it can't be done." Bo Bennett

"Childhood obesity is best tackled at home through improved parental involvement, increased physical exercise, better diet and restraint from eating." Bob Filner

"We're raising our children the way we raise calves for veal—keep them in boxes, feed them too much, and allow them no exercise." Rich Killingsworth, *Center for Disease Control and Prevention*

"The most important thing I want to get across is that maintaining weight loss is just hard. It takes a dedication to exercise and eating right most of the time." Trisha Yearwood

"My recipes aren't geared towards women; my books are marketed towards women because women are the biggest market for weight loss, weight management and weight maintenance and for cooking." Bethenny Frankel

"The measure of self-assurance is how deeply and sincerely interested you are in others; the measure of insecurity is how much you try to impress them with you." Mark Goulston

"Suicide is a permanent solution to a temporary problem." Phil Donahue

"When one realizes that his life is worthless he either commits suicide or travels." Edward Dahlberg

"Life is only a long and bitter suicide, and faith alone can transform this suicide into a sacrifice." Franz Liszt

"A diet changes the way you look. A fast changes the way you see." Lisa Bevere

"Instead of looking outside of ourselves and counting potential enemies, fasting summons us to turn our glance inward, and to take the measure of our greatest challenge: the self, the ego, in our own eyes and as others see us." Tariq Ramadan

"Start the practice of self-control with some penance; begin with fasting." Mahavira

"When you don't have food in your life, just for a day, it makes you realize you're lucky to have it the next day. So the day after fasting, the music that comes out will be very joyous." Chris Martin

"Fasting is, first and foremost, an exercise for identifying and managing adversity in all its forms. With faith, in full conscience, fasting calls women and men to an extra degree of self-awareness." Tariq Ramadan

"Periodic fasting can help clear up the mind and strengthen the body and the spirit." Ezra Taft Benson

"I fast for greater physical and mental efficiency" Plato

"If you do not have control over your mouth, you will not have control over your future." Germany Kent

"Life is never made unbearable by circumstances, but only by lack of meaning and purpose." Viktor Frankl

"To love oneself is the beginning of a lifelong romance." Oscar Wilde

"Your subconscious mind is paying attention to how you treat yourself." Sam Owen

"Self-care has become a new priority – the revelation that it's perfectly permissible to listen to your body and do what it needs." Frances Ryan

"There are days I drop words of comfort on myself like falling leaves and remember that it is enough to be taken care of by myself." Brian Andreas

"The most powerful weapon on earth is the human soul on fire." Ferdinand Foch

"Be who you are and say what you feel, because those who mind don't matter, and those who matter don't mind." Bernard M. Baruch

"Sometimes you have to lose all you have to find out who you truly are." Roy T. Bennett, The Light in the Heart

"An arrogant person considers himself perfect. This is the chief harm of arrogance. It interferes with a person's main task in life—becoming a better person." Leo Tolstoy

"Self-help is not a magic pill. You can read books, and listen to podcasts, but changing is hard. All change is hard at first, messy in the middle, gorgeous at the end." Robin Sharma
"Lose an hour in the morning, and you will be all day hunting for it." Richard Whately

"Every day is a new opportunity. You can build on yesterday's success or put its failures behind you and start over again. That's the way life is, with a new game every day, and that's the way baseball is." Bob Feller

"There is an incredible power that comes from surrounding yourself with communities in which you feel small among them, and they look at you like a giant." Sekou Andrews

"I was trying to daydream but my mind kept wandering." Steven Wright

"Anxiety is the hand maiden of creativity." T. S. Eliot

"Creativity requires the courage to let go of certainties." Erich Fromm

"Without deviation from the norm, progress is not possible." Frank Zappa

"Having a high IQ or being intelligent does not mean ADHD is not a disability." Y.T.

"Life is full of beauty. Notice it. Notice the bumble bee, the small child, and the smiling faces. Smell the rain, and feel the wind. Live your life to the fullest potential, and fight for your dreams." Ashley Smith

"Be sure what you want and be sure about yourself. Fashion is not just about beauty, it's about a good attitude. You have to believe in yourself and be strong." Adriana Lima

"Love yourself. It is important to stay positive because beauty comes from the inside out." Jenn Proske

"Beauty is when you can appreciate yourself. When you love yourself, that's when you're most beautiful." Zoe Kravitz

"Peace is the beauty of life. It is sunshine. It is the smile of a child, the love of a mother, the joy of a father, the togetherness of a family. It is the advancement of man, the victory of a just cause, the triumph of truth." Menachem Begin

"Everything has beauty, but not everyone sees it." Confucius

"No matter how plain a woman may be, if truth and honesty are written across her face, she will be beautiful." Eleanor Roosevelt

"When you do something noble and beautiful and nobody notices, do not be sad. For the sun every morning is a beautiful spectacle and yet most of the audience still sleeps." John Lennon

"Youth is happy because it can see beauty. Anyone who keeps the ability to see beauty never grows old." Franz Kafka

"That's always seemed so ridiculous to me, that people want to be around someone because they're pretty. It's like picking your breakfast cereals based on color instead of taste." John Green

"To be beautiful means to be yourself. You don't need to be accepted by others. you need to accept yourself." Thich Nhat Hanh

"Modeling isn't for the faint of heart, you have to really want it and work hard for it." Liris Crosse

"Modeling is about fantasy, getting people to buy into a lifestyle and a vision." Liris Crosse

"For beautiful eyes, look for the good in others; for beautiful lips, speak only words of kindness; and for poise, walk with the knowledge that you are never alone." Audrey Hepburn

"Example is the school of mankind, and they will learn at no other." Edmund Burke

"Don't worry that children never listen to you; worry that they are always watching you." Robert Fulghum

"Modeling is the best because you have to look hot, which comes easy to me, you know. I'm blessed with that." Ashton Kutcher

"With modeling, you pose. You want to look your best all the time. With acting, you have to be aware of the camera, but the more you show your imperfections, the better you're going to be." Diane Kruger

"Modeling is silent acting." Arizona Muse

"I believe in miracles. At the age of 13, I was on holiday in Moscow with my mother. It was the only trip I took in my whole childhood. We stepped off a metro train and were approached by a talent scout who told me that she wanted to sign me to her modeling agency." Olga Kurylenko

"As a person, I am someone who wants to give my best in every take. I wouldn't say it was easy for me to get into the industry because I come from a background where no one has been in films. But I do believe if you work hard, you will get noticed. Modeling gave me that courage to stand in front of the camera." Pooja Hegde

"Beauty's easy. Modeling is not just about being pretty." Tyra Banks

"What I love the most about modeling is that it opens you a lot of different doors of opportunities and takes you to many different places, which then put you in touch with various people and cultures." Karolina Kurkova

"Modeling teaches you to be completely conscious of the camera. Acting is being unconscious of it." Phoebe Cates

"Imagine for yourself a character, a model personality, whose example you determine to follow, in private as well as in public." Epictetus

"The difference between the girls today and models of the past is that we are not only interested in fashion: we are going in so many different directions at once. We work harder -- at night and on weekends. On the modeling profession." Claudia Schiffer

"Modeling is the most powerful of all teachers!" John G. Miller

"The womb from which you emerge determines your fate to an enormous degree for most of the seven billion people in the world." Warren Buffett

"The best decisions aren't made with your mind, but with your instinct." Lionel Messi

"You can overcome anything, if and only if you love something enough." Lionel Messi

"I start early and I stay late, day after day, year after year. It took me 17 years and 114 days to become an overnight success." Lionel Messi

"Friends and good manners will carry you where money won't go." Margaret Walker

"Respect for ourselves guides our morals; respect for others guides our manners." —Laurence Sterne

"Life is short, but there is always time enough for courtesy." Ralph Waldo Emerson
"Do nothing secretly; for Time sees and hears all things, and discloses all." Sophocles

"The power of community to create health is far greater than any physician, clinic or hospital." Mark Hyman

"You can't exercise your way out of a bad diet." Mark Hyman

"Don't get me wrong, I admire elegance and have an appreciation of the finer things in life. But to me, beauty lies in simplicity." Mark Hyman

"People look for retreats for themselves, in the country, by the coast, or in the hills . . . There is nowhere that a person can find a more peaceful and trouble-free retreat than in his mind. . . So constantly give yourself this retreat, and renew yourself." Marcus Aurelius

Dedication

to Mahatma Gandhi.

Foreword

It is a great honor to write the foreword for *Self-Care: Stay Younger and Live Longer*. Professor M.S. Rao has co-authored this book with his wife, M. Padmavathy. He is an international management thinker, keynote speaker, and award-winning author. He is known as the father of "Soft Leadership" globally. I admire his vision to build one million students as global leaders by 2030.

This book shares the authors' years of experience in health, fitness, food, nutrition, cooking, modeling, and beauty. It explores self-care and explains leading a healthy lifestyle. It defines the perfect day and implores to build character to become a champion. It explains attitude, encourages participation in physical activities and events, and advises making fitness an integral part of life. It emphasizes eating a variety of foods to stay healthy. It lists the foods to eat to boost your memory power. It calls you to eat to live, not live to eat. It has many tips, tools, and techniques to help you live longer.

Toward the end, it elaborates on the causes, effects, and remedies for depression. It has tools and techniques to help prevent unhealthy thoughts to build a happy and peaceful world. It explains the connection between depression and technology. It outlines healthy habits to help you have a better life. It reminds us that preventing depression is better than experiencing it. It implores parents to provide education and character to their children instead of sharing their wealth with their children and calls upon them to prepare their children to face the challenges in life.

This book is written in a conversational tone. Each word in this book is a pearl. The ideas and insights are well-punched. It is a practical book packed with action. It is one of the best books I have read on life leadership. You can gift this book to your friends, and they will thank you forever for caring about them. I wish I had had this book long ago. I highly recommend this book for a deserved place on your leadership bookshelf.

Garry Ridge
Chairman of the Board
& CEO WD-40 Company

Preface

"The doctor of the future will no longer treat the human frame with drugs, but rather will cure and prevent disease with nutrition." Thomas Edison

Welcome to *Self-Care: Stay Younger and Live Longer*. This book outlines self-care and implores you to be the active driver of your life. It advises you to become the best version of yourself. It defines the perfect day and implores you to build character to become a champion. It explains attitude, encourages to participation in physical activities and events, and advises to make fitness an integral part of life. It emphasizes eating a variety of foods to stay healthy. It unveils the advantages of fasting and outlines tools and techniques to check obesity. It unfurls the foods to eat to boost your memory. It advises you to be image-conscious and offers tools and techniques to become a successful model. It calls you to eat to live, not live to eat. It outlines tips, tools, and techniques to stay younger and live longer.

This book elaborates on the causes, effects, and remedies for depression. It offers tools and techniques to prevent suicidal thoughts to build a blissful, peaceful, and prosperous world. It explains the connection between depression and technology. It outlines healthy habits to ensure your mental health and achieve greatness. It reminds us that preventing depression is better than experiencing it. It implores parents to provide education and character to their children instead of sharing their wealth with their children and calls upon them to prepare their children to face the challenges in life. It concludes not to get excited with successes and dejected with failures, but to be level-headed to enjoy peaks and valleys in life.

Thank you from the bottom of our hearts. We hope you enjoy the book!

**Professor M.S. Rao PhD
and M. Padmavathy**

Authors' Note

While all attempts have been made to verify the information provided in this publication, neither the authors nor the publisher assumes responsibility for errors, omissions, or contrary interpretations of the subject matter herein.

The publisher and the authors of the book are not associated with any product or vendor mentioned in this book. None of the companies referenced within the book has endorsed the book. Some names and details have been changed to protect identities.

No content provided in this book, or provided through the links to websites, regardless of date, should ever be used as a substitute for direct medical advice from your doctor or other qualified clinician.

Acknowledgments

Writing a book is never a solo project. We are deeply indebted to many people whose expertise, wisdom, and encouragement kept us going.

We thank **Dr. Abe Khoureis** for his commitment, positive attitude, and professionalism in the publication of this book. Also, we thank all those behind the scenes, editors, production staff, and copy-editors, who have helped bring this work to life.

We would like to thank our coaching clients, who are among the most fantastic leaders. We have learned far more from them than they have learned from me.

We express special thanks to all our readers who graciously took time off from their busy schedules to write to us, share their views, and offer feedback on our books.

1 – Practice Self-Care

"The secret of health for both mind and body is not to mourn for the past, nor to worry about the future, but to live the present moment wisely and earnestly. There are only two mistakes one can make along the road to truth: not going all the way, and not starting." —Gautama Buddha

Throughout my life, I have prioritized my health and enjoyed regular visits to the gym. When I was 15 years old, I started to run since my dream was to join the Indian Air Force and serve my nation. Although I was underweight and short in height, with health issues including asthma, I went to a nearby playground and ran regularly to achieve physical fitness as per the requirements of the military. Through hard work and persistence, I achieved basic fitness and joined the Indian Air Force at the age of 18. After joining, I underwent rigorous military training, improved my height a little bit, and achieved my physical fitness. Whenever and wherever I had an opportunity, I went to the gym in the Indian Air Force units to do the workout. After leaving the service, I continued going to the gym regularly. So I am a fitness freak and a health-conscious person. I joined as a faculty member in an educational institution to shape students as

leaders. I acquired my Ph.D. in soft skills in 2011 and became a professor. I started to
author books after I became a faculty member and continued authoring books because I got a positive response from my publishers and readers. I have published 55 books in various categories, including personality development, success, gender, learning, leadership, and executive coaching. One day, when I was going to the gym, an idea flashed into my mind to author a book on health and fitness. I believe that I am the right person to author a book of this genre to benefit readers. Subsequently, my wife, M. Padmavathy came on board as she is an image consultant, expert chef, and beautician. We included those aspects. Now the book is in your hands, outlining health, wealth, food, nutrition, cooking, modeling, and beauty. Welcome to *Self-Care: Stay Younger and Live Longer*.

When you want to help others, you must help yourself first. When you want to serve others, you must take care of yourself because only when you are healthy will you be able to lead well with heart and soul to serve others and make a difference in their lives. In this introductory chapter, we will discuss self-care, which is the first step to building a healthy world.

What is Self-Care?

"Rest and self-care are so important. When you take time to replenish your spirit, it allows you to serve others from the overflow. You cannot serve from an empty vessel." — Eleanor Brownn

Self-care is not about being selfish but it is to take care of yourself first and lead from the front to serve others. Self-care can be defined as the conscious endeavor to rest and reflect to recharge your batteries physically, mentally, emotionally, and spiritually. Your self-care depends on four pillars—physical, mental, emotional, and spiritual. With the increased technology, people emphasize more on earning their livelihood and staying ahead of others to accomplish their financial goals and objectives. In this process, they forget to set and accomplish their personal and social goals, thus losing their health and landing in health issues in the later parts of their lives. Hence, it is essential to emphasize work-life integration to enable them to lead their personal, professional, and social lives successfully.

Advantages of Self-Care

"Almost everything will work again if you unplug it for a few minutes, including you." Anne Lamott

There are innumerable advantages to emphasizing self-care. Some of them include increased self-awareness, enhanced emotionally, mentally, physically, and spiritually, increased self-esteem, increased productivity and performance, increased self-confidence to overcome challenges, leading from the front, and adding value to others.

The people who emphasize self-care are confident in handling the challenges. They are passionate, persistent, and patient. They are creative and productive. They emphasize work-life integration, balance their personal, professional, and social lives, and provide meaning to their lives.

Tips to Emphasize Self-Care

"With every act of self-care, your authentic self gets stronger, and the critical, fearful mind gets weaker. Every act of self-care is a powerful declaration: I am on my side, I am on my side, each day I am more and more on my side." Susan Weiss Berry

Identify what you want in your life and explore yourself. Set your goals accordingly. Focus on your dreams. When you have your dreams, you engage your mind creatively and productively. Take time to read books, go to the gym, or travel around to unwind yourself. Break your bad habits and acquire healthy habits. You are in this world for a unique reason. Understand this fact and avoid comparing with others. Here are some tips in your arsenal to ensure self-care.

- Pursue your passions and hobbies. Acquire new skills and abilities. Write a gratitude journal.

- Eat food on time. Eat the right foods. Avoid junk food and emotional eating. Sleep well. Take a nap for 10 to 20 minutes to recharge your batteries.

- Keep your stress levels low. Handle it effectively. Do meditation. Spend your time alone to reflect. Remember that solitude is fortitude. Practice gratitude.

- Avoid multitasking. Do one thing at a time. Complete one task successfully and move to another task to execute it effectively.

- Don't compare with others. You are a gift from God, and appreciate this fact and focus on yourself.

- Convert your negative energy into positive energy.

- Don't get addicted to social media. Use it judiciously. Remember, social media is not the real world. It is an imaginative world filled with artificial information.

- Connect with like-minded people to share your emotions and feelings. Meet your relatives and friends periodically to bond with them.

- Take the weekend off to a different location with your family. Enjoy vacation periodically.

- Avoid thinking about your unpleasant past and worrying about your unpredictable future. Instead, think about the present.

- Wed spiritualism to introspect and take feedback.

- Participate in non-profits to connect with people and add value to others.

- Don't wait for an auspicious day to take care of yourself. Instead, start today to take care of yourself.

Some people fail to eat food on time due to their busy schedules. They focus more on their work and less on themselves. At times, competition compels them to neglect their health to stay ahead of the race. But it hurts in the long run. They realize later that they searched for stones by leaving gems at home. They realize their mistakes when the health issues surface at a later stage of their life. Hence, it is essential to care for oneself to keep fit and healthy, overcome challenges effectively, and achieve success.

Be an Active Driver of Your Life

> "Caring for your body, mind, and spirit is your greatest and grandest responsibility. It's about listening to the needs of your soul and then honoring them." Kristi Ling

We are living in a fast-paced world. You must balance everything to lead your life with purpose and meaning. You are gifted with one life, and you must learn how to lead successfully by prioritizing your needs properly. When you want to be significant and serve others, you must focus on your self-care. Unless you are healthy, you will not be able to serve others. Unless you emphasize self-care, you will not be healthy. Hence, emphasize self-care to stay fit and healthy to serve others. To conclude, self-care is the first step to leading from the front to serve others.

> "And in the end, it's not the years in your life that count. It's the life in your years." Abraham Lincoln

2 – Describe Your Perfect Day

"Life isn't just about taking in oxygen and giving out carbon dioxide." Malala Yousafzai

I am a morning man. I wake up at 4 AM every day. I thank God for gifting me one more day for sharing my knowledge with the world free and making a difference. I drink a lot of water. I brush my teeth and go to the washroom. I start writing. At this time, my creative juices start flowing. My mind comes up with new ideas and insights.

I take up one chapter to write about the book. I write whatever comes to my mind about the topic. I capture my ideas without looking into grammar because I edit them at the end. In the middle, I do lots of revisions on the draft.

My wife Padmavathy, wakes up after 5 AM every day and gives me dry fruits—pistachios, walnuts, cashew nuts, almonds, and dates. I eat them. She gives me a spoonful of honey. She prepares tea with milk and serves me. She is an expert in making tea and an expert chef. I am blessed with a beautiful and brilliant wife with a positive attitude. She is amicable and adjustable without any complaining or whining. I enjoy taking tea and resuming my writing. After writing around 4 hours approximately, I take breakfast and go to the gym by walk and it takes one hour to reach and return from the gym. I do a heavy workout in the gym as I am a fitness freak. I started going to the gym when I was 15 years old with a passion to serve my nation. I served in the Indian Air Force. I read a newspaper in the gym for 15 minutes and talked to a few people to identify their unique strengths and inspire them. It takes a minimum of 2 hours to do the workout in the gym and walk every day. After I return home, I take a bath and pray to God. I research in my passionate areas. I deliver keynote conferences and training programs if there are any. If I don't have any such opportunities, I focus on my writing.

I take lunch in the afternoon with my wife and sons. I am emotionally connected with my wife and two sons. I am a homebird and a family man.

I take a nap in the afternoon. After the nap, my mind becomes fresh to write, and I edit what I had written in the early morning. I identify triggers and research them. I check emails and respond to my publishers, friends, and followers. I have different email IDs for different tasks, and I check my emails at least once a day. I share articles, interviews, and books on social media platforms. I view some videos on triggers and training programs and update myself.

In the evening, my wife serves me fruit to eat. After eating and chatting with my wife, I resume my research and writing. At night, I chat with my wife about the developments in the day as she watches television every day. We plan the tasks to be executed the next day. Before

I go to sleep, I plan what to write the next day morning. I give commands to my subconscious mind to become the President of India. I go to bed at around 10 PM.

This is my perfect day. If there are any distractions and disturbances, I manage them effectively to get back to my routine life.

Conclusion

"A day is a day. It's just a measurement of time. Whether it's a good day or a bad day is up to you. It's all a matter of perception." Donald L. Hicks

To conclude, my perfect day includes writing books, sharing knowledge free of charge with the world, coaching others, adding value to others, and building a better world. Life is great.

"I think in the heart of every human being there burns an ember of hope that warmly entices us to believe everything will eventually come together into one perfect day, and that potentially the hours in this day will stretch on indefinitely. And so we live our lives in hopeful anticipation, dreaming and praying to reach this wondrous day, while in the process, we miss out on the anxious affair that life truly is. Life is not perfection; it is everything else. We must taste and experience heartaches and trials to feel the genuine joy that comes from enduring them well. We then move on, wiser and more capable of charity—this being pure love and the reason for life's trials altogether." Richelle E. Goodrich, Slaying Dragons

3 – Be the Best Version of Yourself

"Try to be the best version of yourself." Sara Sampaio

Every person must take feedback and learn continuously to grow as a better person, but few actually do it. Growth is a natural process, but most people remain in their comfort zones. They don't take any initiative to update and become better versions due to various reasons, including fear of failure and criticism. Life is a process from cradle to grave with improvement in all spheres. In this chapter, we will discuss the tools and techniques to become the best version of yourself to add value to yourself and the people around you.

Tips to Become the Best Version of Yourself

"You are unique. You have different talents and abilities. You don't have to always follow in the footsteps of others. And most importantly, you should always remind yourself that you don't have to do what everyone else is doing and have a responsibility to develop the talents you have been given." —Roy T. Bennett, *The Light in the Heart*

Understand what you can control and cannot control. Control only what you can with the internal locus of control. Accept the reality of what you cannot control. Create a circle of healthy friends, talk to them, observe different situations, and explore ways to upgrade your

SELF-CARE: STAY YOUNGER AND LIVE LONGER

skills, abilities, and knowledge regularly. Listen to motivational videos and lectures to stay inspired. Join the non-profit to make a difference in the lives of others. Here are some tips to become the best version of yourself.

- Write down two main tasks you want to do every day and execute them effectively.

- Don't deviate from your core goals and objectives. Stay focused and clear.

- Limit mental masturbation and master your time management.

- Contribute your best in assigned roles and responsibilities. Emphasize excellence, not perfection.

- Read good books. Journal regularly and reflect on them. Take feedback to improve yourself.

- Learn, unlearn, and relearn to stay relevant.

- Lead a healthy lifestyle. Practice gratitude.

Robin Sharma offers the following tips to have a good life: Take daily voyages into awe and regular adventures into wonder. Dedicate time to personal mastery; it will increase your self-love. Celebrate private joys. Look for everyday magic and joy. Don't delay finding peace. Display kindness. Have a coffee at a nice place. Listen to joyful music every day. Be around flowers and nature—they raise your frequency.

Visit art galleries. Read fine books. Eat fantastic food. Bless your money. Bless your body. Avoid bad people. Stay away from drama queens and negativity kings.

Robin Sharma unveils that getting up early is the mother of all habits. If you start your morning well, you will have a great day, weeks, months, years, and decades. You can't have a world-class life if you don't start your mornings well. It's essential to spend three hours every morning on personal development. He wakes up at 5 am, no matter where in the world he might be. He lies in bed for some time, recites a mantra, visualizes, prays, and practices deliberate gratitude. He journals in his diary. He doesn't write on his smartphone. He advises not to take shortcuts.

Conclusion

"The seduction of complacency and an easy life is one hundred times more brutal than a life where you go all in and take a stand for your dreams. World-class life begins where your comfort zone ends." Robin Sharma

Character is built from childhood. Character is a collection of various aspects, including attitude, personality, behavior, habits, principles, practices, ethics, and etiquette. Habits can be acquired and avoided over some time by people depending on their personal preferences, time factors, and association with others. You can lead your life with purpose and meaning only when you become the best version of yourself.

To become the best version of yourself, you must change your habits to build your character to lead a meaningful and happy life.

"Never be bullied into silence. Never allow yourself to be made a victim. Accept no one's definition of your life, but define yourself." Harvey Fierstein

4 – Build Your Character to Become a Champion

"Vision gets the dreams started. Dreaming employs your God-given imagination to reinforce the vision. Both are part of something I believe is necessary to build the life of a champion, a winner, a person of high character who is consistently at the top of whatever game he or she is in."
Emmitt Smith

Most parents think of offering wealth to their children to lead a prosperous life. Most educational institutions think of equipping their students to equip with the knowledge to ensure employment. Most societies think of providing resources to their citizens to achieve overall development. They must all think of building an impeccable character to make them champions in life. In this high-tech world, most people think of achieving success at any cost to outsmart others. Some of them go to the extent of achieving success by hook or crook. Some of them cut corners to achieve success. What is essential is to build character to become champions in their lifetime. In this chapter, we will discuss building character in people to enable them to provide meaning to their lives.

When you want to become a champion, you must assess your strengths and weaknesses, leverage your strengths, and guard from your weaknesses. It is observed that most people focus too much on overcoming their weaknesses rather than on leveraging their strengths, which is counterproductive. Instead, they must focus on their strengths and capitalize on them to excel as champions.

Build Your Character

"Intelligence plus character – that is the goal of true education. The complete education gives one not only the power of concentration but worthy objectives upon which to concentrate." Martin Luther King Jr

The character cannot be formed in a comfort zone. The character can be formed when people enter into complex situations and crises. How people react to situations and the environment by keeping others' interests above their interests reflects their true character. It is easy to talk about building character in letters, but it is difficult to follow in spirit, especially when things go out of control. Anyone can helm the affairs when the sea is smooth, but the real leadership emerges when the sea is rough. Michael Josephson remarked, "Character is both formed and revealed by how one deals with everyday situations as well as extraordinary pressures and temptations. Like a well-made tower, the character is built stone by stone, decision by decision." Building character is easier said than done.

Building character is not the responsibility of educational institutions alone. It is the responsibility of parents, relatives, family, society, and above all, individuals themselves. Several factors influence building character, such as heredity, environment, and situation. Additionally, how people approach resolving issues reflects their character. Michael Josephson remarked, "Character is made up of core moral principles called the six pillars of character: trustworthiness, respect, responsibility, caring, fairness, and citizenship. Each of these virtues is independently important, but together they provide the foundation for a worthy life."

Become a Champion

"Good character is not formed in a week or a month. It is created little by little, day by day. Protracted and patient effort is needed to develop good character." Heraclitus

Building character is a continuous process. It takes time, effort, and interest to build character. Anne Frank remarked, "Parents can only give good advice or put them on the right path; the final forming of a person's character lies in their own hands." People must invest conscious efforts to build their character because it is the character that lasts, not charisma.

Character is one thing that differentiates between ordinary and extraordinary people. It is the character that makes people champions in their lifetime. It is the character that makes them immortal in the annals of history. Hence, emphasize character, not charisma. Emphasize ethics, not wealth. Above all, add value to others to excel as a champion. To conclude, create a roadmap to build your character to become a champion in your life.

"Try not to become a person of success but rather try to become a person of value." Albert Einstein

5 – Improve Your Attitude

"Our visit to this planet is short, so we should use our time meaningfully, which we can do by helping others wherever possible. And if we cannot help others, at least we should try not to create pain and suffering for them."
—Dalai Lama

In this world of distractions due to information overload, it has become a big challenge to focus our minds on positive aspects and constructive activities. Sometimes we waste our precious time mentally and physically due to distractions arising out of technology. We must understand our priorities and learn how to focus on them religiously. In this chapter, we will discuss attitude and tips to stay focused clearly on goals and objectives.

Improve Your Attitude

"Whenever you conflict with someone, there is one factor that can make the difference between damaging your relationship and deepening it. That factor is attitude."
William James

With the right attitude, you can achieve anything and everything in the world. In the 20th century, intensive research was done to identify the reasons behind successful people. It was unveiled that attitude made them stand out from others globally. Your attitude determines your altitude of success.

Globally, attitude, knowledge, and skills are widely discussed. Among them, it is the attitude that plays a crucial role in acquiring knowledge, skills, and abilities. When you discuss personality, attitude, and behavior, it is the attitude that plays a crucial role in improving your personality and behavior. When you talk about hard skills and soft skills, it is the soft skills that matter more, and attitude is the crucial element to acquiring soft skills. In a nutshell, it is the attitude that makes your life 100 percent successful and meaningful.

The three components of attitude are what you feel, think, and do. Your education, environment, and experience determine your attitude. Hence, ensure that you acquire ethical education and are surrounded by positive people to enable you to have positive experiences in life.

The negative attitude results in self-doubt, low self-esteem, ill health, stress, bitterness, and resentment. Anyhow you are going to invest your energies, then why not invest your energies in building a positive attitude instead of a negative attitude? To acquire a positive attitude, you must think positively, surround yourself with positive friends, develop a can-do mentality, appreciate others, and above all, live in the present.

Tips to Focus on Constructive Activities

"I have learned from experience that the greater part of our happiness or misery depends on our dispositions and not on our circumstances." Martha Washington

Whenever negative thoughts pop up in your mind, affirm repeatedly that you were born with certain gifts in life. Leverage those gifts to grow and add value to others. Here are some tips in your arsenal to focus on your goals and objectives to achieve amazing success in your life.

- Engage your mind constructively on your goals and activities. Fix some time daily on them. Avoid multitasking.

- Create an environment with the right kind of noise. Surround yourself with friends who are positive, constructive, and healthy. Create a team of strong connections who are experts in creating ideas and taking their ideas into execution.

- Share your personal feelings and emotions with your trusted friends. Avoid wearing your emotions on your sleeve.

- Follow your passions and hobbies. Leverage the technology.

- Breathe in and breathe out for a few seconds to divert your mind. Remember to breathe with your stomach and through your nose. Do meditation and yoga.

- Engage your mind in household chores. Connect with your family members. Spend considerable time with them.

- Hold your mind continuously on your goals for 21 seconds to enable you to stay focused on your goals.

- Undertake much bigger challenges and focus on them to resolve them.

- Understand the fact that people are quickly glued to negative aspects rather than the positive aspects.

- Stop complaining, criticizing, and condemning others. Take responsibility for your actions.

- Focus more on your strengths and less on your weaknesses. Focus more on ideas and less on individuals and issues.

- Overcome your apprehensions and anxieties. Stay away from superstitions. Look at the door that is open, not the closed one. Have an open mind to resolve issues. Find out what is bugging you. Explore solutions to overcome them.

- Travel to unwind. Take a vacation to break from your negative thoughts. Go on a pilgrimage if you are a religious person.

- Don't compare with others. You are unique and a gift from God. Nobody can be like you, and you cannot be like anybody in the world.

- Be magnanimous to help others and add value to them.

- Maintain a gratitude journal to express your gratitude every day.

- Consult a psychologist to seek professional advice.

Strengthen your subconscious mind. Give positive commands to your subconscious mind 30 minutes before you go to bed. These commands will have a positive impact on your mind and improve your personality, attitude, and behavior.

Grow your potential by concentrating on your passionate goals; improving yourself continually; forgetting your unpleasant past, living in the present; and focusing on the future.

Conclusion

"We can't stop the waves, but we can learn to surf." Jonathan Kabat-Zinn

Don't visualize negative events in life. Don't exaggerate them

overly. Don't make a mountain out of a molehill. Remember that everyone has challenges in life. You are not an exception.

Understand this fact and enlighten yourself to lead a pleasant and peaceful life. In real life, there are takes and retakes, but in real life, there are only takes, no retakes. You are on a short visit to this planet. You are gifted with one life. Ensure that you lead your life constructively to provide meaning to your life.

> "Ninety percent of those who fail are not defeated. They simply quit." Paul J. Meyer

6 – Lead a Healthy Lifestyle

"People who laugh actually live longer than those who don't laugh. Few people realize that health actually varies according to the amount of laughter." James J. Walsh

A healthy lifestyle is essential to lead a happy and exciting life. The rapid growth in technology has brought threats and opportunities to humankind. It has connected humans globally and brought comfort to them. At the same time, it has posed health challenges to humans, including anxiety and depression. Therefore, there is an urgent need to emphasize a healthy lifestyle to ensure the happiness and progress of the human race in the right direction. Hence, we will discuss leading a healthy lifestyle in this chapter.

A healthy lifestyle includes eating sensibly with the right foods in the right proportions, exercising your body, associating with positive people, adding value to yourself, and making a difference in the lives of others. There are three symptoms of good health, such as good appetite, free motion, and sound sleep. If people possess them, they are leading a healthy life. Here are some tips in your arsenal to lead a healthy lifestyle.

- Express your gratitude early morning when you get up from bed and take feedback every day before you go to bed.

- Take proper care of your body. Eat right. Exercise every day. Sleep adequately.

- Begin your day with real food, such as fruits or a handful of nuts, or dry fruits such as figs and dates. You can follow this up with tea or coffee after 30 minutes.

- Eat with your family members. Avoid gadgets and television viewing while eating. Chew food properly to ensure effective digestion. Avoid taking excessive salt because it can cause strokes and heart attacks.

- Brush your teeth at least twice a day, preferably after meals. Limit your consumption of sugary and acidic foods and avoid using your teeth for anything other than chewing food.

- Drink moderately. Remember that heavy drinking can cause high blood pressure, irregular heartbeat, or sudden death from heart failure. Avoid drinking on an empty stomach.

- Maintain a correct posture because it can play a vital role in keeping your bones and joints aligned so that the various muscles in your body are used correctly. It also reduces the rate at which your joint surfaces wear out and decreases the stress on the ligaments that hold the joints of your spine together.

- Acquire a positive, right, and strong attitude. Surround

yourself with positive people. Spread positivity. Inspire the people around you. Add value to others.

- Set short-term and long-term goals. Focus on them. Be productive, patient, and persistent.

- Follow your passion. Acquire new skills and abilities. Read great books. Read one book a week.

- Create multiple sources of income to achieve financial stability and security. Be frugal, but don't be cheap. Save for a rainy day.

- Avoid carrying emotional baggage.

- Use technology wisely. Shed outdated technology and wed modern technology. Avoid information overload.

- Maintain a gratitude journal and express your gratitude every day.

- Be simple, humble, and noble.

Maintain a positive body language. Respect others' views and opinions. Agree to disagree. Avoid interfering with others' issues.

Lead Your Life on Four Pillars

"Lack of activity destroys the good condition of every human being, while movement and methodical physical exercise save it and preserve it." Plato

To summarize, eat right and exercise regularly. Drink 8 glasses of water a day. Sleep 8 hours every day. Work 8 hours five days a week. Connect with your family members emotionally. Travel to unwind. Follow your passion. Pursue a hobby. Participate in nonprofits. Add value to others to build a better world. Make a difference. Pass on your baton to the next generation. Leave your legacy. To conclude, lead your life based on four pillars—health, wealth, love, and happiness to provide meaning and leave your legacy.

"You must be very patient, very persistent. The world isn't going to shower gold coins on you just because you have a good idea. You're going to have to work like crazy to bring that idea to the attention of people. They're not going to buy it unless they know about it." Herb Kelleher

Reference

https://news.harvard.edu/gazette/story/2018/04/5-healthy-habits-may-increase-life-expectancy-by-decade-or-more/

7 – Make Fitness an Integral Part of Your Life

"To keep the body in good health is a duty; otherwise, we shall not be able to keep our mind strong and clear." Buddha

With the increased life expectancy, there is increased interest shown in health globally. People are more conscious about their health than ever before. A few years ago, wealth was accorded importance over health. However, there is a shift in the mindset of people globally toward health because they have started to realize that health is wealth. Hence, in this chapter, we will discuss the importance of health and wealth, taking people from happiness to prosperity.

Importance of Health

"When health is absent, wisdom cannot reveal itself, art cannot become manifest, strength cannot be exerted, wealth is useless, and reason is powerless." Herophiles

Health can be defined as the well-being of an individual physically, mentally, emotionally, intellectually, occupationally, socially, and spiritually to lead a happy and prosperous life. When your health is sound, you will have a healthy heart, mind, and body. You will have increased life expectancy. You will be able to socialize with people of all age groups and cultures due to your confidence and emotional intelligence. You will lead a quality and meaningful life. You will be resilient to overcome stressful situations and achieve amazing success in all spheres of your life.

Fitness and Its Advantages

"Lack of activity destroys the good condition of every human being, while movement and methodical physical exercise save it and preserve it." Plato

Fitness is the ability to meet the demands of the environment and execute tasks and activities effectively. Fitness can be divided into health-related fitness and skill-related fitness. Cardiovascular fitness, strength, muscular endurance, flexibility, and body composition fall in the category of health-related fitness, while agility, balance, coordination, speed, reaction time, and power fall in the category of skill-related fitness. There are many advantages of physical fitness and nutrition. It reduces high blood pressure, depression, anxiety, fatigue, risk of premature death, risk of developing diabetes, risk of developing high cholesterol, and body fat. It builds and maintains healthy muscles, bones, and joints; enhances work, recreation, and sports performance; improves overall well-being; and leads a healthy and happy life.

Fitness is different from physical activity. Physical activity is about anything that gets you moving. It helps you engage productively and lead a healthy lifestyle. It improves your bone mass, immunity, mental health, and cardiorespiratory fitness. It checks diabetes, enhances weight control and lifespan, and reduces cancer risk. It is better to be active than to be sorry for your health. When you are active, you can do your things. You don't have to depend on others. You can check obesity. Your body permits you to do things by yourself. It increases your self-esteem and self-confidence. It has been proven that exercise can help improve memory problems. According to the American Medical Association (AMA), "Exercise improves cognitive (memory) function in older adults with subjective and objective mild cognitive impairment." The flow of blood into your whole system can work wonders. More serious brain problems—Alzheimer's disease and related dementias may also show considerable improvement.

Here are some advantages of strength training exercises. It increases your strength, functional capacity, and body density. It prevents injury and ensures better balance and stability. Above all, it improves your self-esteem and self-confidence. Observe the following tips to be physically active. Take the stairs instead of the elevator. Do gardening. Play with kids and pets. Park the car farther away from your destination. Do exercises while watching TV.

How to Get Started?

"The last three or four reps are what make the muscle grow. This area of pain divides the champion from someone else who is not a champion. That's what most people lack, having the guts to go on and just say they'll go through the pain no matter what happens." Arnold Schwarzenegger

To get started, consult the doctor to check your present health condition. Examine your current health habits. Set your fitness goals. Join the gym. Hire an expert trainer to achieve your fitness goals. If you find it difficult to go to the gym, come out of your comfort zone and go to the gym for 21 days continuously to get used to going to the gym regularly. If you find it challenging to go to the gym, connect with like-minded people who go to the gym regularly. They motivate you to go to the gym every day. You can improve your health and build connections, too.

Your Diet Plan

"Want to learn to eat a lot? Here it is: Eat a little. That way, you will be around long enough to eat a lot." Anthony Robbins

Before your workout, take a light snack and stay hydrated. Your regular diet must be low in fat, cholesterol, and sodium. Avoid taking large meals. Take meals in a limited quantity but ideally between 4 to 6 times a day. Ensure that your diet is a proportionate blend of carbohydrates, proteins, and fats. Carbohydrates are the chief source of fuel; proteins repair the muscles and enhance growth; and fats offer an extra fuel source for your muscles. You must eat right to remain healthy and fit. Eat raw vegetables because the skin of such vegetables contains vitamins. You must eat a variety of foods such as fruits, vegetables, nuts, grains, meat, fish, and dairy.

Create Your Fitness Program

"We are what we repeatedly do." Aristotle

Here are some fundamental elements of fitness. Cardiovascular fitness gives you the ability to exercise your entire body for long periods. Strength fitness gives you the amount of force your muscles can produce. Muscular endurance fitness gives you the ability to use your muscles many times without tiring. Flexibility fitness gives you the ability to use your joints fully through a wide range of motion.

When we speak about physical exercise, it is not just jogging, weight-lifting, or some popular fad. Exercise and physical activity must have four components: endurance, strength, balance, and flexibility. We must advocate a balanced approach so that we get the full benefit and a feeling of physical wellness.

Endurance can be achieved through aerobic activities like walking or jogging, which increase your breathing and blood circulation. Do cardiovascular activities for at least 30 minutes a day. Do strengthening exercises six days a week. Lift dumbbells and weight machines. Do pull-ups, push-ups, squats, and arm dips on a bench. Take breakfast regularly.

Drink plenty of water before starting your exercises and moderate water during and post exercises. Learn a new sport

to keep yourself physically active and fit, and build leadership qualities.

Create your fitness program in such a way that you do exercises every day to different parts of your body to ensure the overall fitness of your body. Give rest to your body once a week to enable it to recharge effectively. Don't do the same activities every day. Reshuffle your activities to enable the body to take rest for the exercised portions and ensure fitness for other parts to achieve overall physical fitness. While doing workouts, emphasize strength-building and endurance-building activities. Blend moderate and vigorous activities proportionately. Avoid fitness-related injuries such as overuse injuries and traumatic injuries. Overuse injuries arise due to continuous stresses on tendons, bones, and ligaments during workouts. Traumatic injuries arise due to sudden or violent activities during a workout. Hence, it is advisable to do your workout under the guidance of an expert trainer if you are a novice.

Make Fitness Your Lifetime Commitment

Our moods can either lift us into emotional heights or take us into the depths of depression that could be paralyzing. Exercise can help you give zest to a tired life and bring zing into your being. Physical activity stimulates various brain chemicals that make you feel happier and more relaxed. It will boost your confidence and improve your self-esteem. To conclude, make fitness your lifetime commitment and ensure that it becomes an integral part of your life to stay healthy forever

"Physical fitness is not only one of the most important keys to a healthy body, it is the basis of dynamic and creative intellectual activity." J.F. Kennedy

8 – Participate in Physical Activities and Events

"Never underestimate the power of dreams and the influence of the human spirit. We are all the same in this notion: The potential for greatness lives within each of us." Wilma Rudolph, winner of 3 Olympic gold medals I have had a keen interest in participating in physical activities and events since childhood. When I was 15 years old, I had a dream of joining the Indian Air Force to serve my nation. I went to the gym regularly to achieve physical fitness as per the standards of the Indian Air Force. Although I was short in height with a lean physique and health issues, including asthma, I actively participated in physical activities and events wherever I lived.

I joined the Indian Air Force when I was 18 years old and went to the gym apart from acquiring rigorous military training, whenever I found time. Once, I participated in a marathon event with my two sons in Chennai. We believed in participating, not in winning any medals. We enjoyed participating in activities and events. We participated in a swimming competition in 2007, and I won a gold medal. I moved to different locations in India when I served in the Indian Air Force, but the passion to participate in events never died. In 2018, I decided to participate in a 10K run in Hyderabad to enjoy the event.

But I was not able to enroll in it. Since I am a researcher and author, I did a little research to understand the fundamentals of the event.

Dos and Don'ts to Run Successfully

"All you need is the courage to believe in yourself and put one foot in front of the other." Kathrine Switzer

Consult the doctor before participating in the event. Be passionate about running. Don't do it just because others are doing it. If you are persuaded that you can pull it off, enter the race. Create a blueprint to proceed with your running plan. Work hard, smart, and wisely to win the race. Create time logs. Prepare a diet plan. Follow them religiously. Eat plenty of carbs the night before the event. Eat enough calories and drink a good quantity of water. To be a successful runner, it is ideal to have a lean and healthy body. Here are some tips to run successfully.

- Adopt a visualization technique. Visualize mentally that you are winning the race.

- Strengthen your subconscious mind before going to bed every day that you are winning the race.

- Follow the '21-day' principle. You may find it difficult to run initially. Hence, force yourself hard to run for 21 days, and you will be amazed to find running from 22 days onwards, and you will enjoy running.

- Don't have a big meal before the event. Eat bananas to fuel your body.

- Avoid taking tea before the event.

- Take adequate water two hours before the event.

- Warm up your body before the event. It prepares your muscles and prevents injuries.

- Understand your body first and start running accordingly.

- Sip a little water while running.

- Inhale through the nostrils and exhale through the mouth to prevent the throat from getting dry.

- Don't fold your shoulders. Don't run with a heel landing on the ground. Instead, land on the midsole of your foot.

- Avoid taking either a long or a short stride. Instead, take an average stride. In the military, the soldiers are trained to take an average stride while marching forward to bring uniformity, uniqueness, and rhythm.

- If you are a novice and find it challenging to run, you can run and walk and resume your running. Gradually, you can stop walking and start running continuously. In this way, you can get used to running.

- Count your minutes, not miles, during the event.

- Start slow at the start line and end with energy in the finish line. Run slowly and steadily in the beginning. When you approach the goal, invest all your energy to accelerate your speed to win the race. Bill Bowerman, renowned University of Oregon coach, remarked, "It's better to run too slow at the start than too fast and get into oxygen debt, which is what 99.9 percent of runners do. You have to learn pace."

- Rest well before the event.

You can run faster if you have a strong body and proper posture, and adopt the right running strategy and techniques. You must focus on coordination, mobility, agility, flexibility, stretching, strengthening, dynamic, and mental preparation to win the game.

Conclusion

"The biggest mistake that new runners make is that they tend to think in mile increments—1 mile, 2 miles, 3 miles. Beginning runners need to think in minutes, not miles." — Budd Coates, four-time U.S. Olympic Marathon Trials qualifier/coach

To win in a running or marathon event, you must have a systematic activity and a healthy diet. You must work hard consistently and raise your bar constantly to stand out from others. You must avoid smoking and drinking alcohol to excel as a successful athlete and a winner. To conclude, follow the tips, tools, and techniques to participate in events and activities in your area to keep your body agile, active, and healthy.

"Toeing the starting line of a marathon, regardless of the language you speak, the God you worship, or the color of your skin, we all stand as equals. Perhaps the world would be a better place if more people ran." Dean Karnazes

9 – Participate in Sports and Games Regularly

"Sport is a preserver of health." Hippocrates

Playing sports and participating in games regularly keeps you healthy and happy. Globally, children are encouraged to participate in sports and games to enable them to become fit physically and active mentally. When children are active physically, they can concentrate effectively on education. Hence, educational institutions emphasize curricular and extracurricular activities to groom students as well-rounded personalities. In this chapter, we will discuss the significance of sports and games in becoming fit mentally and physically to become a complete person.

The Significance of Sports and Games

> "Sports build good habits, confidence, and discipline. They make players into community leaders and teach them how to strive for a goal, handle mistakes, and cherish growth opportunities." Julie Foudy

People think that sports and games are the same. However, there is a difference between them. Sports may be individual activities, while games are group activities with players. There are innumerable advantages associated with sports and games. They play an important role in the body, mind, and soul. They encourage you to become active physically and mentally. They help you maintain mental balance amid hope and despair. They break monotony and boredom. They help you discover your strengths and weaknesses. They improve your blood circulation. They strengthen your bones and help coordination, balance, and flexibility. They give you a dash of endorphins and help you overcome your anxiety and stress. They give you enjoyment and freshen your mind. They build a positive attitude and outlook on life. They build your self-esteem and self-confidence. They develop emotional intelligence to get along with others. They develop team spirit, leadership, and communication skills.

They build hard and soft skills. They teach you the art of winning and the craft of bouncing back from failures successfully. They build tenacity and resilience. They prepare you to take success and failure equally. They build a killer instinct and teach you to be patient and persistent. They build great habits that make you successful. They build your character. Billie Jean King remarked, "Sports teach you character, they teach you to play by the rules, they teach you to know what it feels like to win and lose teaches you about life." Hence, participate in sports and games to lead your personal, professional, and social life happily.

Sports and games help you make decisions quickly, enhance sociability, work collaboratively, and prepare you to overcome challenges in life. They help you be accountable and responsible. They manage your time effectively and help you to understand what you can control and what you cannot control. They make you practical and realistic. They make you simple and humble. There is a promising career in sports and games if you work hard and sincerely for some years. You will earn money, fame, and awards, and become a celebrity. You can also become a brand ambassador and explore other entrepreneurial opportunities, including setting up your own sports institution or academy.

Conclusion

> "The power of the human will compete and the drive to excel beyond the body's normal capabilities is most beautifully demonstrated in the arena of sport." Aimee Mullins

Playing outdoor games improves your physical and mental health, while playing indoor games improves your memory power and enhances your concentration. Sports and games ensure a sound mind in a sound body. Education is incomplete without them. Hence, encourage sports and games at an early age in life to excel as a successful person.

> "Sports is human life in microcosm." Howard Cosell

10 – Eat a Variety of Foods to Stay Healthy

"Let food be thy medicine, thy medicine shall be thy food." Hippocrates

A healthy mind starts with a healthy stomach. We can safely claim today that what is good for the gut is good for the heart and also for the head. The message is to eat right to enable your heart to be fit and your head to be right. In this chapter, we will discuss a variety of foods, their importance, and eating a variety of foods.

Food and Categories

> "Your diet is a bank account. Good food choices are good investments." Bethenny Frankel

You can group food into five categories, such as carbohydrates, fruits and vegetables, proteins, dairy, and fats and sugars. The main function of carbohydrates is to give you energy. If you eat more than required your body stores it as fat. Fruits and vegetables provide your body with the minerals and vitamins it needs to maintain good nutrition. Protein helps your body to repair itself and assists with growth and the smooth running of your body parts.

The diary provides your body with vitamin A and vitamin D; however, some dairy products can have a high fat content. Your bodies use fats and sugars for energy; however, you need very little fats, and it is better to get your energy from carbohydrates. Large amounts of saturated fats can cause heart disease, which is the biggest killer in adults today, because their arteries become clogged up with fat deposits.

Food and Its Significance

"A healthy diet is a solution to many of our health-care problems. It's the most important solution." —John Mackey

Carrots, sweet potatoes, liver, butter, and margarine contain vitamins that fight infections and improve your vision. Citrus fruits, juices, and dark green vegetables contain vitamins that maintain healthy bones and teeth and reduce stress. Fortified milk, liver, tuna, and eggs contain vitamins that ensure growth, form bones and teeth, and help absorb calcium. Grains, green leaf vegetables, saturated fats, and vegetable oils contain vitamins that guard red cells and help the metabolism of free fatty acids. Liver, wheat bran, peas, soybean oil, and potatoes contain vitamins that help blood clotting.

Proteins help muscle tissue develop and function. Protein is needed to make hair, skin, nails, muscles, organs, blood cells, nerves, bone, and brain tissues, enzymes, hormones, and antibodies. Vitamins are complex organic compounds found in small amounts in most foods. They do not contain calories and therefore do not provide energy. Minerals do not contain calories but are important to many bodily functions. There are two groups of minerals: major minerals and trace minerals. All food provides calories. All calories provide energy. However, calories that do not come with vitamins, minerals, fatty acids, amino acids, and fiber are called "empty calories." Empty calories give you energy without nutrients. Table sugar and alcohol are examples of empty calories. Eating too many foods with empty calories can cause health problems. Here is a list of foods and their importance.

- Milk products give you calcium. Calcium builds strong teeth and bones. Even though we think of milk as a drink, it is a food.

- Foods from the meat, fish, and beans group give you protein. Protein builds strong muscles. You should eat 2 servings of the meat, fish, or beans group a day. It is best to eat only 2 to 3 servings of red meat a week. Fish and fish oils help keep your brain healthy and alert.

- Meat and fish are best cooked on the barbecue or a grill so that the fat drains off. Before cooking meat, ensure you cut off as much fat as you can.

- Eat more tomatoes as lycopene, a powerful antioxidant found in them, could help protect against the kind of free radical damage to cells that occurs in the development of dementia.

- Carrots help to cleanse the body, assisting the liver in flushing out toxins. It reduces bile and fat in the liver. The fiber present in carrots helps bowel movement and cleans out the colon.

- Olive oil can encourage the food to move quickly in the digestive tract, naturally improving bowel movements. The oil also promotes the strengthening of our bone structure. Olive oil has shown itself as a powerful metabolism booster, making us feel good overall.

- Coconut water is known to have the same electrolyte levels as human plasma and has even been used for plasma transfusions.

- Honey reduces ulcers and other gastrointestinal disorders. It can be used to reduce coughs and colds, heal wounds and burns, treat allergies, and fight various infections. If you are feeling lazy and low, try honey. Spread it on hot toast or chapatti ... and replace the sugar in your tea with it for a refreshing surge of energy. Honey, being anti-bacterial and anti-fungal is known for its incredibly long shelf-life.

- Turmeric offers a unique color and flavor. It contains anti-inflammatory properties that are used to treat digestive illnesses such as diarrhea, stomach bloating, and liver problems. It is also an antioxidant that is used to treat various pain and emotional conditions, including headaches, depression, menstrual problems, as well as cancer.

- Colorful plant foods provide an abundance of cancer-fighting & immune-boosting nutrients!

- Mushrooms have been known right from ancient civilizations and were reserved for royalty. In Egypt, they were thought to be strengthening and so given to soldiers.

Tips to Eat the Right Diet

> "Food is an important part of a balanced diet." — Fran Lebowitz

Taste is one of the five senses sight, smell, sound, taste, and touch. Taste buds are receptors that detect the 5 known elements of taste perception: sour, bitter, sweet, and savory. We have 2,000-10,000 taste buds! If you load up your palate with salt, then all the other tastes may be missed.

You need an adequate and varied diet to stay healthy. Healthy eating improves your life and lowers blood pressure, blood sugar, and blood cholesterol, and the risk of heart attack and stroke. Hence, make healthy food habits by reducing simple carbohydrates, fried foods, and unhealthy fats; and replacing them with more vegetables, fresh fruits, grains, nuts, and beans. Try different kinds of foods. Here are some tips to eat the right diet.

Be aware of what you are eating. Keep a food journal. Write down what you eat, how much you eat, when you eat, and why you eat. Eat more vegetables and some fruits such as apples and pears. Diets low in refined carbohydrates work best.

Choose whole grain bread, cereals, pasta, and rice, and keep intake moderate. Eat more fish, poultry, beans/lentils, eggs, and less red meat. Avoid saturated and trans fats and use more plant oils-canola oil, olive oil, peanut oil, healthy margarine, mayo, and salad dressings. Eat two portions of fish a week, one of which should be oily fish that includes mackerel, salmon, trout, sardines, pilchards, and fresh tuna. Eat milk and dairy foods in moderate amounts. Eat foods containing fat and sugar in small amounts.

Make it a goal to try one new fruit or vegetable every week. Eat at least five portions every day. Ensure that you are satisfied after eating, not stuffed. In a nutshell, make changes in foods and eat carefully; plan healthy meals; and minimize saturated fats, sodium, and sugar. Remember that diet, exercise, and a positive attitude help lead a happy and healthy life.

For older people, it is ideal to eat foods that are nutrient-dense rather than energy-dense, including eggs, lean meats, fish, liver, low-fat dairy foods, nuts and seeds, legumes, fruit and vegetables, whole grain bread, and cereals. They must spend some time outside each day to boost vitamin D synthesis for healthy bones. They must limit foods that are high in energy and low in nutrients, such as cakes, sweet biscuits, and soft drinks. They must choose foods that are naturally high in fiber to encourage bowel health.

Conclusion

> "The food you eat is making you sick, and the agencies that are providing you with guidelines on what to eat are giving dangerous advice with devastating health consequences. You can change that today." Dr. William Davis

Most chronic diseases are caused by wrong food habits and related nutritional deficiencies. Modern-day consumer styles have damaged our bodies to such an extent that the medical industry is thriving because of our reckless eating habits. Hence, understanding various foods and their advantages helps you choose the right foods to ensure great health. To conclude, eat a balanced diet with a variety of foods to stay healthy and happy.

> "Insanity: Doing the same thing over and over again and expecting different results." Albert Einstein

Reference

https://www.betterhealth.vic.gov.au/health/healthyliving/food-and-your-life-stages

11 – Boost Your Memory with the Right Foods

"A sharp memory depends on your total number of brain cells, the smooth flow of communication between the cells, and the health of cells." Joy Bauer, *author of Food Cures and Nutrition expert*

There are several ways to slow down forgetfulness when you get older. Adopting certain practices and eating the right foods can boost your memory and prevent dementia. In this chapter, we will discuss the types of foods to eat to boost your memory.

Tips to Boost Your Memory

> "A brain filled with well-nourished neurons enables you to think and remember more clearly." Joy Bauer

Research shows that foods including oily fish, coconut oil, eggs, walnuts, dark chocolates, green tea, ginkgo, rosemary, dandelion greens, avocado, jicama, kale, spinach, almonds, pumpkin seeds, chickpeas, Indian gooseberry, Brahmi, cinnamon, honey, kimchi, asparagus, banana, and berries boost your memory. Here are some tips to boost your memory. Sleep well. Drink plenty of water. Exercise regularly. Go for a massage. Avoid excessive sugar and alcohol. Drinking juices will decrease Alzheimer's disease risk. Drink grape juice. Eat apples. Take a glass of wine a day. Above all, turn things into pictures to remember people.

Lisa Evans, in her article, *Sharpen Your Memory with Brain-Healthy Foods* in Entrepreneur, suggests eating six foods to keep your grey hairs from affecting your grey matter: beets, fish, berries, lean protein, walnuts, and coffee. She explains that beets regulate heartbeat; fish maintain brain cell health; berries prevent brain cell breakdown; lean protein improves cognitive skills; walnuts improve memory scores; and coffee sharpens focus.

Foods including barley, oatmeal, cherries, walnuts, almonds, sweet potatoes, kale, bananas, red peppers, chia seeds, acai, quinoa, camu, moringa, sprouts, carrots, and brown rice increase your endurance. Foods including watermelon, strawberries, blueberries, oysters, seafood, nuts, figs, chili peppers, apples, ginger, wild salmon, oats, garlic, nuts, tuna fish, pomegranate, arils, beets, spinach, avocado, asparagus, red wine, steak, mustard, red bell peppers, brazil nuts, black-eyed peas, halibut, pesto, pumpkin seeds, and dark chocolate increase your sexual stamina. What is good for your heart is good for your lower body. Apart from eating the right foods, you must reduce stress, stay away from bad habits, pay attention to your partner, and be active to boost your libido.

When you want to enjoy exciting sex, count the amount of ecstasy you receive, not time. Count quality, not quantity. A Journal of Sexual Medicine study reports that the average time couples spend bumpin' and grindin' ranges from three to 13 minutes. Other research reveals that most women want "sexy time" to last between 15 and 25 minutes—not for hours like some people might think. Regardless, nothing bad can come from going at it a bit longer!

Some people use tablets and pills to increase their sexual power in bed. Instead, they must eat the right foods and adopt the right practices to increase their sexual power and pleasure in bed. Enjoying exciting sex maintains a healthier weight and a stronger immune system. Hence, include libido-boosting foods on your plate to keep your sex drive happily humming.

Metabolism

Metabolism helps convert food into energy. It slows as one ages. It increases when your body is exposed to extreme temperatures. Usually, men have a higher metabolism than women. Women who are pregnant have a faster metabolism. Exercising hard burns more calories and increases metabolism.

Invest in Aerobic Exercises

Doing aerobic exercises regularly helps keep you healthy and happy. Aerobic exercises must not be confused with anaerobic exercises such as weightlifting or sprinting, which involve quick bursts of energy with maximum effort and minimum time. Several exercises fall in the category of aerobic exercise, such as walking, jogging, running, cycling, swimming, rowing, dancing, and boxing. There are innumerable advantages of aerobic exercise. It increases your breathing and heart rate. It helps you keep your heart, lungs, and circularity system healthy. It adds strength to your muscles and increases endurance.

Your heart beats approximately 60-80 times per minute at rest, 100,000 times a day, more than 30 million times per year, and about 2.5 billion times in a 70-year lifetime! Every beat of your heart sends a volume of blood (called stroke volume -- more about that later), along with oxygen and many other life-sustaining nutrients, circulating through your body. The average healthy adult's heart pumps about 5 liters of blood per minute. Below is a list of aerobic activities with the approximate number of calories burned per hour for a 150-pound individual.

Aerobic class: 450-500
Bicycling (outdoor): 540-620
Bicycling (stationary): 480-540
Cross-country skiing: 530-630
Dancing: 300-350
Gardening: 270-300
Hiking: 400-480
Jogging: 530-630
Jumping rope: 650-800
Running: 650-750
Skating: 470-550
Swimming: 400-480
Tennis: 470-550
Volleyball: 200-240
Walking (regular pace): 150-200
Walking (fast pace): 250-300

Hence, invest daily for 30 minutes in aerobic exercise to stay healthy and happy.

Conclusion

"I eat very clean, healthy food at all times because I'm very focused on keeping myself in shape." Jodi Lyn O'Keefe

There are several reasons why people become vegetarians and vegans. They are concerned about the environment, want to improve their health, decrease world hunger, and prevent animal cruelty. Food habits are your personal choice. But ensure that you eat food not only to please your taste buds but also to achieve great health.

> "When it comes to food and memory, fish should be the star of the show." Joy Bauer

References

https://www.entrepreneur.com/article/226179

https://www.alzheimers.net/foods-that-induce-memory-loss/

https://www.eatthis.com/healthy-foods-that-increase-sexual-stamina/https://www.medicinenet.com/aerobic_exercise/

12 – Drink Water Adequately

"Water is the driving force of all nature." Leonardo da Vinci

Water makes up more than two-thirds of the human body's weight. A mere 2% drop in our body's water supply can start making us feel dehydrated, and this is one of the most common causes of daily fatigue. So, our wellness depends much on the intake of water. A healthy human being living in ideal conditions, not in the unbearable heat or cold, and not exerting oneself too much, can only survive for about 3 to 5 days without water. In this chapter, we will discuss the significance of drinking sufficient water.

Here are some facts and findings about water. An individual must drink 6-8 cups of water daily and more if participating in sports or exercising. Water is the most critical nutrient for sustaining life. Two-thirds of the human body is water. Water makes up 60% of your total body weight and 70% of your muscles; raw meat is about 75% water, and fruits and vegetables up to 95% water. It may take us weeks to starve, but only a very few days to dehydrate. About 3/4 of our water is contained within individual cells.

Advantages of Water

> "When the well is dry, we'll know the worth of water." Benjamin Franklin

Water doesn't have any calories. There are innumerable benefits of drinking adequate water. It hydrates your body and gives you energy. It flushes toxins out of your body, decreases wrinkles, and glows your skin. It improves your appearance and enhances your beauty. It increases your metabolism, burns more fat, and ensures weight loss. It regulates your body temperature, eliminates waste, and protects your joints and organs. It allows your kidneys to remove toxins from your body. It prevents you from cramps and sprains. It protects your tissues, spinal cord, and joints. It helps create saliva, ensure digestion, and prevent constipation. It helps excrete waste through perspiration, urination, and defecation. It improves your mood and enhances your physical performance. It fights illness and keeps you away from diseases.

Proper hydration helps keep joints lubricated and muscles more elastic to keep you agile during your daily routines. When your muscles are energized, you feel the whole body tingling. Since your brain is mostly water, drinking plenty of water helps you think, focus, and concentrate effectively. You will be more alert, your muscles will be energized, and your energy levels will be higher. When you're getting enough water, urine flows freely. If you are the kind who drinks too little, you may be at higher risk for kidney stones.

So keep drinking water.

Myths about Water

"Water used to be fresh, pure, and drinkable; now the water has lots of local matter and bacteria." Claudine Sierra

There are a lot of myths about how much fluid we should have, but Faisal Abdalla2 suggests, "Your body weight in kilograms divided by 30=your suggested daily intake in liters. And then add another 350 ml for every 30 minutes that you work out. For instance, if you weigh 90kg, start by drinking three liters.

Andrea Cannistraci writes, "Instead of costly and non-environmentally friendly bottled water, I request carafes of ice water. Yes, it's good for the environment, but it's also important to stay hydrated when choosing a healthy lifestyle. Humans should drink at least 1 gallon of water per day. And when spending time in a desert environment or high altitude, water consumption is more important than ever."

Tips to Increase Your Water Intake

> "Thousands have lived without love, not one without water." W.H. Auden

You can include water in your daily routine by consuming fruits such as apples, bananas, watermelon, grapefruit, and strawberries; vegetables such as celery, lettuce, radish, zucchini, spinach, tomato, and eggplant; and milk, yogurt, and soup. Here are some tips to increase your water intake.

- Take a sip of water every time you pass the water fountain.

- Carry a water bottle with you wherever you go.

- Have a glass of water, unsweetened tea, fat-free/skim milk, or 100% fruit juice with your meals.

- Place a glass of water by your desk side to have a "water break."

- Choose a cup of yogurt or fruit for a snack.

Drink magnetized water daily because it regulates the cells of your body. When water is subjected to a strong magnetic field, there are certain changes in its properties, and such water is known as "magnetized water." You can magnetize water within 12 hours by placing one bottle or glass on the North Pole (red) and the other on the South Pole (blue) and mixing them.

Conclusion

> "Pure water is the world's first and foremost medicine." Slovakian Proverb.

Don't drink excessive water. Drink only adequate water. Both overhydration and dehydration lead to headaches. Don't drink water for the sake of drinking. Drink only when you are thirsty. Don't drink water until the color of your urine is clear. Pale yellow urine is a sign of good health. An ideal way of drinking water is to take 5-6 glasses of water as soon as you get up in the morning, even before you brush your teeth. Do this three times daily if you are suffering from arthritis or rheumatism, To conclude, drink water after you wake up from your bed as it enables you to activate internal organs; 30 minutes before taking your meal as it enables you to digest; before taking bath as it enables you to lower your blood pressure; and before going to bed to prevent heart attacks.

"Water is critical for sustainable development, including environmental integrity and the alleviation of poverty and hunger, and is indispensable for human health and well-being." United Nations

References
https://www.mirror.co.uk/lifestyle/health/having-positive-mental-attitude-key-12714940
https://www.prevuemeetings.com/spark-blog/flip-the-script/integrate-wellness-meeting-like-pro/
https://www.hsidn.org/uploads/6/6/8/7/66873073/water_powerpoint.pptx
http://www.klientsolutech.com/importance-of-water/

13 – Overcome ADHD

> "It is better to be high-spirited even though one makes more mistakes than to be narrow-minded and all too prudent." Vincent Van Gogh

If you behave impulsively, it could be a sign of attention deficit/hyperactivity disorder (ADHD). If you find it hard to pay attention to your education or tasks and interrupt others when others speak to you, it could be a symptom of ADHD. If you feel restless mentally and are constantly active, it could be a signal of ADHD. Research shows that ADHD is prevalent in some people globally. In this chapter, we will discuss the signs, signals, symptoms, and solutions for ADHD.

Signs, Symptoms, and Signals of ADHD

> "I am not absentminded. It is the presence of mind that makes me unaware of everything else." G.K. Chesterton

ADHD is a medical condition where an individual has differences in brain development and brain activity that affect attention, the ability to sit still, and self-control. It can affect children at school, at home, and in friendships. It is more common in people with learning difficulties. Some of the causes of ADHD include premature birth, low birth weight, genes, drinking alcohol, smoking cigarettes, and brain injuries. Dr. Barnhill says, "Foods treated with organophosphates for insects seem to cause neurologic-based behavior problems that mimic ADHD." People with ADHD are hyperactive, impulsive, and rash in their attitude and approach. They start work quickly but lose focus quickly. They are poor listeners. They may forget their daily routines and chores. They become distracted easily by unrelated thoughts and are often inundated with too many ideas. They talk nonstop and are impatient to wait for their turn to talk during conversations with others. They don't sit in one place and find it difficult to be quiet. They brood over the same things for a long time. They get frustrated easily. They find it difficult to gel with others. They cannot control their anger. They cannot concentrate while reading. They daydream a lot.

Solutions to Overcome ADHD

"In the power of fixing the attention lies the most precious of the intellectual habits." Robert Hall

Consult a healthcare professional to identify whether you have ADHD. If you have been diagnosed that you have ADHD, remember that it is not a major disease. Here are some solutions to overcome it. Step out of your comfort zone and engage effectively to accomplish your goals and objectives. Do meditation daily. Be passionate, patient, and persistent. Acquire new skills and abilities. Focus on your work rather than its outcome. Believe in karma. Focus on being a better professional than on career advancement. Lead from behind. Care about the success of your team members. Avoid taking any medicines. Instead, change your diet and your lifestyle. Join nonprofits and social activities to add value to others. Make a difference because it gives you great joy and happiness apart from engaging your mind constructively.

A 2015 study published in the Journal of Abnormal Psychology found that 30 minutes of exercise before school can help kids with ADHD focus and manage moods. It can even eliminate or decrease the need for stimulant medications used to treat symptoms. Exercise boosts the brain's neurotransmitters—chemicals that many individuals with ADHD run short on. It primes the brain for learning, and environmental enrichment helps to make important connections happen. Hence, exercise regularly. When you are systematic, organized, and consistent, you can easily overcome ADHD. Hence, lead a disciplined, systematic, and organized life to overcome ADHD.

Eat the Right Foods

Eat high-quality calories. Eat foods that are rich in fiber and protein to stay alert, calm, and focused. Eat the right foods containing Omega-3s, Zinc, Iron, Magnesium, Vitamin C, Valerian, Melatonin, Ginkgo, and Ginseng. However, ensure that they don't have any side effects. Omega-3s are believed to be important in brain and nerve cell function. A new study3, conducted at Göteborg University, in Sweden, concluded that daily doses of omega-3s—found in cold-water, fatty fish, such as sardines, tuna, and salmon—reduced ADHD symptoms by 50 percent. Dr. Sven Ostlund followed a group of ADHD children aged 8-18 who took fish oil daily. Within six months, there was a noticeable decrease in ADHD symptoms in 25 percent of the children. Avoid excessive intake of sugar. Avoid exposure to certain foods including milk, chocolate, soy, wheat, eggs, beans, corn, tomatoes, grapes, and oranges. Drink plenty of water.

Conclusion

> "ADHD is not about knowing what to do, but about doing what one knows." Dr. Russell Barkley

Don't treat ADHD as a stigma. There are many eminent and highly successful people, including Abraham Lincoln, John F. Kennedy, Albert Einstein, Thomas Edison, Norman Schwarzkopf, Andrew Carnegie, Bill Gates, Richard Branson, Michael Jordan, Vincent Van Gogh, Britney Spears, Jim Carrey, Michael Phelps, and Justin Timberlake lived and thrived with ADHD. They succeeded because they were self-aware and leveraged it creatively. To conclude, ADHD can be cured through self-awareness, education, medication therapy, or a combination of treatments.

"To invent, you need a good imagination and a pile of junk." Thomas Edison

References

https://www.nimh.nih.gov/health/publications/attention-deficit-hyperactivity-disorder-adhd-the-basics/index.shtml

https://kidshealth.org/en/parents/adhd.html

https://www.additudemag.com/what-is-adhd-symptoms-causes-treatments/

https://www.additudemag.com/adhd-diet-nutrition-sugar/

14 – Detoxify Your Body, Mind, and Soul Periodically

> "For the first time in the history of the world, every human being is now subjected to contact with dangerous chemicals, from the moment of conception until death." Rachel Carson, Silent Spring

Globally, detoxification is widely discussed in health circles. It is practiced widely in developed nations and less in less developed nations. Climate change and the modern work environment have thrown several health challenges, leading to increased emphasis on detoxification. In this chapter, we will discuss detoxification and its significance.

What is Detoxification?

"A systemic cleansing and detox is the way to go after each holiday. It is the key to fighting high blood pressure, heart disease, cancer, and other health-related illnesses." —Lee Haney

Detoxification is the process of removing toxins from your body. It is essential when we have high toxins in our bodies. People become sick when their bodies build up waste and contain toxins. The food we eat is adulterated, the water we drink is contaminated and the air we breathe is polluted. Hence, the importance of detoxification is more necessary than ever before. Detoxification is recommended periodically based on the body, personality of the individual, and the environment.

Advantages of Detoxification

"Drink warm water with lemon first thing in the morning. It's a good way to detox and alkalize your body. Valentina Zelyaeva

There are innumerable advantages of detoxification. It strengthens your immunity system and helps in getting rid of toxins from your body. It cleanses the liver, puts out the fire, helps with weight loss, ensures healthier skin, and achieves better mental health. Here are some ways to flush out toxins from your body. Buy organic food and clean it thoroughly. Increase your fiber consumption. Cut out sweet beverages. Eat more brassicas, preferably. Drink plenty of water. Start your day with lemon water. Drink green tea. Exercise regularly. Eliminate toxic substances. Decrease stress in your life.

Foods such as eggs, oats, onions, garlic, lentils, beans, citrus fruits, and yogurt help you detox naturally. When you detoxify physically, you remove toxins. When you detoxify mentally, you remove negative thoughts and replace them with positive thoughts. When you detoxify emotionally, you forget your unpleasant past and overcome your emotional baggage. When you detoxify spiritually, you focus more on the soul than the body and mind.

According to a 2016 report published by the World Health Organization (WHO), outdoor air pollution has risen by 8% globally in just the last five years. In a 2012 paper for the National Institutes of Health, Dr. David Bellinger hypothesized that 16.9 million IQ points had been lost in children because of everyday pesticide exposure. Both regular drug use (illegal substances and prescribed pharmaceuticals) and regular drinking take their toll on our detoxification pathways, especially on the liver and the digestive system. The National Survey on Drug Use and Health (NSDUH) found that 21.5 million American adults battled substance abuse in 2014.

Conclusion

> "Let's detox our cluttered academic brain. That's what the poet does. People call it daydreaming, detoxing our minds, and taking care of that clutter. It's being able to let in call letters from the poetry universe."
>
> Juan Felipe Herrera

You detoxify physically when you focus on your body, you detoxify mentally when you focus on your mind, and you detoxify spiritually when you focus on your soul. Hence, detoxify periodically to keep your body, mind, and soul active, happy, and peaceful.

"I treat myself pretty good. I take lots of vacations, I eat well, I take supplements, I do mercury detox, I get plenty of sleep, I drink plenty of water, and I stay away from drama and stress." Reba McEntire

Reference

https://thetruthaboutcancer.com/signs-you-need-to-detox

15 – Be Image Conscious

> "The beauty of a woman is not in a facial mode, but the true beauty in a woman is reflected in her soul. It is the caring that she lovingly gives and the passion that she shows. The beauty of a woman grows with the passing years." Audrey Hepburn

Humans want to be approved and recognized by others for their attitude, appearance, personality, and behavior. Most women appreciate being elegant and beautiful. They want to attract the attention of men. Although men want to look smart, they emphasize more on intelligence and machoism. However, we find a few men emphasizing appearance and elegance apart from being intelligent. In this chapter, we will discuss tips to appear elegant, smart, and beautiful.

Tips to Appear Elegant and Beautiful

> "She was beautiful, but not like those girls in the magazines. She was beautiful, for the way she thought. She was beautiful, with the sparkle in her eyes when she talked about something she loved. She was beautiful, for her ability to make other people smile, even if she was sad. No, she wasn't beautiful for something as temporary as her looks.

> She was beautiful, deep down to her soul. She is beautiful." F. Scott Fitzgerald

Everyone is not blessed to be born with an appropriate appearance. Physical appearance is mostly connected with genes. However, you can improve your appearance by adopting certain tips and following certain practices. All that you must do is invest a little money and time in your posture, hair, eyebrows, complexion, teeth, and make-up to improve your beauty. Here are some nuggets to appear elegant, smart, and beautiful.

- Cultivate good habits to boost your confidence.

- Maintain a positive body language. Smile wherever it is appropriate.

- Wear comfortable clothes to suit your body, height, color, and complexion. Understand that certain styles of dresses look better on certain body types and dress appropriately.

- Use makeup carefully. Remember that makeup is an art. Therefore, invest in the right brushes to achieve the desired outcomes.

- Get your eyebrows waxed regularly if you are a woman.

- Wash your face when you return home to keep your skin clean and avoid pimples and blemishes.

- Drink adequate water to stay hydrated and keep your skin glowing and hair healthy. Additionally, water flushes out toxins from your body and keeps wrinkles at bay. If the color of your urine is clear, that means you are adequately hydrated. Remember, not to stick to the "eight glasses a day rule" because the need for water differs from person to person and climatic conditions. Drink coconut water to keep your liver clean.

- Avoid junk food. Eat a healthy diet. Eat moderately. Eat boiled or roasted beets every day. Eat a handful of raw nuts every day. Eat almonds when you feel hungry. Avoid excessive intake of salt to avoid raising your blood pressure. Additionally, when your intake of salt is excessive, your kidneys find it hard to flush out impurities.

- Drink green tea because it is enriched with nutrients and antioxidants. It improves your blood circulation, lowers cholesterol, and improves your skin.

- Drink lemon water every morning. It cleans your system, improves your immunity, enhances your mood levels, clears your skin, and ensures weight loss.

- Rinse your hair with peppermint water. Scrub your body with salt and sour cream. Do mustard hair masks twice a week.

- Do sun salutations every morning. Go for a walk or gym every day for some time to elevate your energy levels. Avoid excessive intake of alcohol. Drink moderately and drink red wine preferably.

In a nutshell, don't worry, be happy. Be positive and healthy. Smile graciously. Appreciate others. Have an attitude of gratitude. Wear clothes within your budget and dress well. Care for your body and maintain it regularly. Visit the beauty parlor to add value. Eat fruits and drink enough water. Sleep well. Have sex regularly. Above all, love yourself to be confident, smart, brilliant, and elegant. Emphasize inner beauty to enhance your external appearance.

In general, women have four body types[1]: apple (top-heavy, with big busts and thinner legs), straight/rectangular (waist and hips are roughly equal, "boyish"), pear (bottom-heavy, with hips significantly larger than bust), and hourglass (equal hip and bust measurements, with a narrow waist). In general, men have four body types too: average (with broad shoulders tapering down to the waist), inverted triangle (athletic, with moderate to heavy muscle definition), rectangular (skinny or narrow in build, with the waist and the shoulders being the same width), or the triangle (a more pronounced midsection with narrower shoulders).

Conclusion

"Some of us teach ourselves and our children to love

the superficial outer; our looks, hair, skin, clothes rather than the greater beauty that resides within, whereas it is that inner beauty that really defines you and who you truly are." Rassool Jibraeel Snyman

Certain aspects are gifted by birth, while certain aspects are cultivated. If you can leverage your inborn gifts and observe certain practices and tips, you can appear attractive, elegant, smart, and beautiful.

"Never lose an opportunity of seeing anything beautiful, for beauty is God's handwriting." Ralph Waldo Emerson

References

http://uk.complex.com/style/2015/04/how-to-dress-for-your-body-type-men/dressing-for-tall-men-dressing-for-short-men http://upstatecouture.com/beauty/10-beauty-tips-how-to-look-more-attractive-in-one-month/

16 – Pursue Modeling as a Career

"The secret to modeling is not being perfect. What one needs is a face that people can identify in a second. You have to be given what's needed by nature, and what's needed is to bring something new." Karl Lagerfeld

Modeling is a highly sought-after profession globally. It is an incredible profession. It is a profession of fantasy where young girls and boys enter to earn name and fame. But it is not as easy a profession as many outside people think. Undoubtedly, it is a lucrative profession but is replete with many challenges and opportunities. If you are passionate about this profession, you must work hard with commitment and excellence to succeed in this industry. There are several myths associated with this industry. In this chapter, we will discuss pursuing modeling as a career to become a successful model.

Merits and Demerits of the Modeling Profession

"Girls interested in modeling need to realize that it's hard work. You can go to a shoot in the morning and not even start shooting until 10 pm—and still be there at 5 am the next day. Then if you still haven't got the shot, you'll have to go back the next day and start again!" —Kate Moss

Every profession has merits and demerits, and modeling is not an exception. The advantages include traveling extensively, meeting great people, building connections, getting handsome remuneration, enhancing your visibility, excelling as a celebrity, and leading a luxurious life. You can also explore other related businesses. The disadvantages include irregular timings, challenging working environments, stressful conditions, and rapidly changing designs and styles. There is a lack of financial stability in this industry. It is like a 'feast or famine'. That means, there will be more money or no money in this profession. This is an insecure profession financially, with fluctuating fortunes. The success rate in this profession is low.

Some models hit the limelight and vanish quickly. There is no longevity in this profession. Be careful about this profession, as there are sex scandals, controversies, and the use of drugs. Therefore, aspiring models must note these aspects. If you are truly passionate about this profession, you must pursue it aggressively.

Challenges and Controversies

"The world of modeling can be hard; just as cruel as it is glamorous." Cindy Margolis

There is a cut-throat competition among models since the opportunities are limited. It takes guts to become a model in this cut-throat, competitive world. You must have a unique mindset, toolset, and skillset to succeed as a model. Remember, a modeling career is highly taxing physically, mentally, and emotionally. Adriana Lima rightly remarked, "Modeling is a tough job, your co-workers are your rivals, and it puts a damper on your perspective of other girls." There are other challenges, including eating disorders among models. There are several controversies associated with this profession, including sexual harassment, blackmail, and exploitation. Fernanda Ly remarked, "I was once shooting a lookbook where the stylist, helping me dress, used this chance to feel my body up much more than necessary and continued to do so throughout the entire shoot. Countless times have I had to undress in undesirable public situations, but even now I can remember the disgusting feel of this man's hands tracing my body." Those who intend to become models must note these aspects and assert themselves to overcome these challenges.

Tips to Become a Successful Model
"One thing that modeling did was that you go to do a different job every day, and you are working with a completely new team of people. You have to learn how to talk to people and how to creatively achieve the same goals. I think it just hones your people skills." Cat Deeley

There are several fields in modeling, such as print modeling, ramp modeling, television modeling, showroom modeling, and endorsement modeling, to name a few. Choose the one that excites you before you enter this profession. There are several types of models, such as fashion models, runway models, commercial models, fitness models, and hand models, to name a few. Here are some tips to become a successful model. Identify your talents and build your skills around them. Shortlist the right agency that is genuine and ethical. Be punctual and professional. Observe ethics and etiquette. Emphasize excellence. Don't take the opportunities for granted. Blend hard skills and soft skills.

Soft skills matter more than hard skills in the modeling profession. You must listen and learn from all sources and manage all stakeholders to accomplish your professional goals. Don't complain, criticize, or condemn others. Be diplomatic to survive in this industry. Be assertive. Avoid offering sexual offers that jeopardize your career in the long run. Don't resort to shortcut methods to reach the top position quickly because it boomerangs finally. Be mentally prepared for frequent rejections. Be passionate, patient, and persistent. Keep financial reserves ready. Remember to start your career as early as possible to build a long portfolio, strong experience, and great connections. Leverage social media to build your leadership brand.

"So many women are having to compromise their physical and often mental health for the advancement of their careers. The boundaries of what a model should be are too black and white, leaving little or no room for error or individuality. Of course, there are wonderful role models like Ashley Graham and Iskra, championing body positivity but the industry's reluctance to stray into the 'middle ground' of sizing is alarming and limiting." Emily Butcher

Conclusion

"I started out modeling at a young age and surrounded myself with different brilliant minds. I have so many people to get educated from, and I've been a sponge." Kellan Lutz

With the entry of more educated women and men entering into this profession, there is more sanctity associated with this profession. Hence, choose this profession, dream big, and work hard, smart, and wisely to become a successful model.

"Modeling is an incredible job for a girl if she approaches it with her head on her shoulders. You travel, you speak to people, and it opens your mind to different things." Anja Rubik

Reference

https://fashionista.com/2017/03/model-fashion-problems-treatment-abuse-health

17 – Explore Stoic Philosophy to Achieve Peace and Happiness

"True happiness is to enjoy the present, without anxious dependence upon the future, not to amuse ourselves with either hopes or fears but to rest satisfied with what we have, which is sufficient." Seneca

With the advent of technology and the Fourth Industrial Revolution (FIR), there is increased volatility, uncertainty, complexity, and ambiguity globally. People find it challenging to predict where the technology will take them to the next level. They are excited with the innumerable advantages arising from automation and artificial intelligence, but they are equally concerned about the threats arising from them. Precisely, humans are caught between peace and prosperity. In this chapter, we will explore stoic philosophy and its relevance in today's world to achieve peace and prosperity.

What is Stoicism?

"Do not seek for things to happen the way you want them to; rather, wish that what happens happen the way it happens: then you will be happy." Epictetus

Stoicism is a way of life. It is the unofficial religion of the Roman world. It is closely connected with mindfulness. It helps you identify what you can and cannot control. It enhances your self-awareness and enlightens your life. It strengthens your self-control, increases your inner strength, and enhances your endurance. It is an amazing therapy against heartache.

Stoicism can be defined as the ability to encounter adversaries and face failures with a cool, calm, collected, and composed demeanor. It is working under pressure with grace. Life throws several curveballs, and people must be ready to face them squarely, which is possible when they adopt Stoic philosophy. The philosophy of stoicism was founded in the 3rd century BC in Athens by Zeno of Citium and practiced by eminent philosophers including Marcus Aurelius, Seneca, Epictetus, Cato, Cleanthes, Hecato, and Musonius Rufus. It is also practiced in the military.

Stoic philosophy is based on the pillars of self-awareness, emotional control, mindfulness, and resilience. Precisely, this philosophy is based on the pillars of character, courage, convictions, conscience, communication, charisma, compassion, consideration, and contribution. There are innumerable advantages of adopting a stoic philosophy. For instance, you differentiate between what you can control and what you cannot control. You make choices wisely. You don't criticize, complain, or condemn others. You become mature, remain calm, and evolve as a philosophical person.

Myths and Truths about Stoics

"Everything we hear is an opinion, not a fact. Everything we see is a perspective, not the truth." —Marcus Aurelius

There are several myths about stoicism and stoicism. For instance, there is a myth that stoics are stone-hearted. The truth is that they have hearts with emotions, egos, and feelings, but they can control and manage their emotions, egos, and feelings internally. They are extraordinary people who don't exhibit their inner emotions and feelings to others. They appear calm like ducks because ducks struggle with their feet beneath the water to stay afloat but appear calm externally.

There is a myth that stoics suppress their emotions, but the fact is that they channel their emotions creatively and constructively to remain calm and composed, irrespective of the outcome. There is a myth that stoicism is a religion. The truth is that stoicism is a way of life and is not connected with any religion. It is a philosophy of living mindfully rather than existing in this world.

Characteristics of Stoic Leaders

"Perform each task at hand with precise analysis, unaffected dignity, human sympathy, and dispassionate justice. Vacate your mind from other thoughts. Perform each action as if it were the last of your life." Marcus Aurelius

Stoics are different, not indifferent to the sensitivities of others' egos, emotions, and feelings and the external environment. Their attitude prepares them for failures and guards them against the arrogance of success. They are silent and resilient, accepting the external realities and controlling and channeling their inner energies to turn the tide in their favor. They are emotionally intelligent and balanced and take both successes and failures equally. They know their limitations and work within the available resources without blaming external forces and factors.

Stoic leaders have a high internal locus of control. They live in the present. They have detached themselves from the desire for an outcome. They emphasize excellence and have an attitude of gratitude. They live with the ground realities and lead a simple and humble life. They expect less and embrace more. They understand that life is full of peaks and valleys and embrace change effectively. They know when to hold and when to fold. They suffer silently to achieve their goals and objectives. They are visionaries and optimistic, and adopt different strategies to accomplish their goals.

However, they are unsure about the duration of their success as they are aware that many things are beyond their control. They remain calm and collected despite encountering adversity after adversity. They internalize their education and experience to spark action with smarter and wiser decisions. They take feedback at the end of each day, journal regularly, and reflect a lot to improve themselves. They enjoy their solitude. They handle conflicts effectively and overcome crises. They can lead all stakeholders mindfully. Precisely, they compare less, criticize less, and consume less. They create more, learn more, and live more.

Scott Christ unfolds 8 important lessons stoic leaders will teach you about being happy. Stoic leaders connect with the world around them. They live in the present moment. They live a life of virtue. They harness the power of their mind. They don't get worked up over stuff that doesn't matter. They stop caring what others think about them. They cultivate strong relationships by doing selfless acts for people they love. They are thankful for what they have and stop worrying about what they don't have. Some of the Stoic philosophers, such as Cato the Younger, influenced leaders including George Washington, John Adams, and Benjamin Franklin. Eminent American leaders, including Thomas Jefferson and Theodore Roosevelt, political thinker John Stuart Mill, and economist Adam Smith, followed stoicism. The leaders who remained stoic in the face of adversity include Abraham Lincoln during the American Civil War, James Stockdale during the Vietnam War, and Lieutenant Michael Murphy during the Afghanistan War.

A Blueprint to be Stoic in Adversity

"The business of life is more akin to wrestling than dancing, for it requires us to stand ready and unshakeable against every assault, however unforeseen." Marcus Aurelius

Here is a blueprint to be stoic in adversity. Understand and appreciate the fact that there is increased volatility, uncertainty, complexity, and ambiguity (VUCA) across the world. Have an internal locus of control. Improve your attitude, personality, and behavior. Leverage your uniqueness. Treat your failures as lessons. Convert your negative thoughts into positive thoughts. Convert your threats into opportunities. Convert your scars into stars.

Lead Your Life Mindfully

> "To be a philosopher is not merely to have subtle thoughts, nor even to found a school…it is to solve some of the problems of life not only theoretically, but practically." Henry David Thoreau

Remember that troubles of the past and anxieties of the future are the thieves of present-day happiness. Hence, live in the present mindfully to lead your life with purpose and meaning. Observe the following nuggets to lead your life mindfully. Decrease your computer screen time. Avoid excessive viewing of TV. Avoid thinking too much about unpleasant experiences. Avoid shopping addiction.

Overcome relationship issues. Don't procrastinate. Avoid clutter physically, mentally, and emotionally. If you view it negatively, life looks full of pain, problems, and challenges. If you view it positively, life looks full of harmony, happiness, and beauty. Hence, view life positively to overcome the challenges and add value to others. Carol Burnett rightly remarked, "Only I can change my life. No one can do it for me."

Explore Stoic Philosophy

> "We should hunt out the helpful pieces of teaching and the spirited and noble-minded sayings which are capable of immediate practical application—not far-fetched or archaic expressions or extravagant metaphors and figures of speech—and learn them so well that words become works." Seneca

Entrepreneurs and leaders encounter unprecedented challenges regularly. Adopting stoicism helps them greatly to overcome their challenges. To summarize, Stoicism is a neglected field in ancient philosophy. Stoic philosophy is relevant in today's world. It is time to understand and adopt it in the current complex world. You cannot change everything in the world, but you can change your attitude by acting towards them proactively to lead a happy and peaceful life. To conclude, explore Stoic philosophy to achieve inner harmony, peace, and happiness

> "That's why the philosophers warn us not to be

satisfied with mere learning, but to add practice and then training. For as time passes, we forget what we learned and end up doing the opposite, and hold opinions the opposite of what we should." Epictetus

References

https://www.lifehack.org/articles/lifestyle/8-important-lessons-stoic-philosophy-will-teach-you-about-being-happy.html

https://dailystoic.com/anthony-long/

https://classicalwisdom.com/philosophy/actionable-philosophy/

https://dailystoic.com/category/interviews/

18 – Eat to Live, not Live to Eat

> "Obesity is a problem that nearly every nation in the world is facing, but there is much that we can do to fix it." Richard Attias

Obesity is a big challenge globally, especially in developed countries, while starvation is a big challenge globally, especially in less developed countries. When people eat more and exercise less, it leads to obesity. However, when people are deprived of food, it leads to starvation. It is a paradox in the global society presently. Jonathan Sacks rightly remarked, "Close to a billion people—one-eighth of the world's population, still live in hunger.

Each year, 2 million children die from malnutrition. This is happening at a time when doctors in Britain are warning of the spread of obesity. We are eating too much while others starve." In this chapter, we will discuss losing weight and fasting periodically to lead an active and exciting life.

Although people are aware of obesity, they eat more due to their cravings. At times, genetic factors are responsible for overeating. Some celebrities undergo liposuction to reduce their fat, which is not advisable. A focus on health rather than illness will save you money and lead a happy life.

How to Lose Weight?

> "By eating many fruits and vegetables in place of fast food and junk food, people could avoid obesity." —David H. Murdock

When energy intake is higher than energy expenditure, you gain weight. In contrast, when energy intake is lower than energy expenditure, you lose weight. Hence, there must be a fine balance between energy intake and energy expenditure. Here are some tips in your arsenal to lose your weight.

- Set SMART goals where SMART is the acronym for specific, measurable, achievable, realistic, and time-bound.Avoid a sedentary life. Increase your physical activities. Exercise every day to build up muscle. Focus on aerobic exercises and strength or muscle endurance exercises. Hire a professional trainer.Decrease your caloric intake. Avoid fad diets because they give short-term, quick outcomes but don't give lasting outcomes.Take quality food to improve your metabolism and genes. Remember that cutting back on calories is not the solution to prevent weight gain.

- Avoid binge eating. Control cravings. There is a thin difference between hunger and craving. Hunger is an acceptable one, while craving is an unacceptable one.

- Drink water 30 minutes before you take your meal. Eat enough healthy food. Eat unprocessed foods. Chew your food properly. Eat slowly to enjoy your food and ensure effective digestion. Take limited meals 4 to 6 times a day. Eat more fruits and vegetables. Digest and absorb it.

- Don't sleep immediately after taking food. Walk around after you take a meal to let the food settle down and digest within the system.

- Manage your stress and sleep well for 8 hours.

- Go slowly and steadily to accomplish your goals. Don't adopt any shortcuts. Work hard to tone down your body. Listen to your body and your trainer.

Here are some more tips to lose weight. Set long-term goals. Improve the nutritional quality of your diet. Make changes in your intake of food. Modify your daily routines towards a healthy lifestyle to ensure a healthy weight. Take a meal only when you are hungry. Avoid the intake of sugars and starches in your food because they reduce your appetite and lower your insulin levels. Enjoy eating protein, fat, and vegetables. Consume low-carb vegetables including broccoli, cauliflower, spinach, kale, brussels sprouts, cabbage, swiss chard, lettuce, and cucumber. Increased physical activity increases the metabolic rate. Avoid excessive alcohol. Avoid a sedentary life. Avoid artificial sweeteners.

Exercise regularly. Sleep adequately. Drink moderately. Avoid drinking beer. Take feedback periodically to measure your progress and modify your activities. Following these tips to lose weight enhances your self-esteem and confidence. You will be able to lead your life with pleasure and confidence. Remember to eat to live, not live to eat.

Why do most Diets Fail?

Most diets fail because dieters are not committed to their health goals. They give up due to their cravings. Hence, dieters must control their cravings and be willing to stick to their health goals consistently. Additionally, dieters often go back to their old habits and practices after accomplishing their goals. Therefore, dieters must continue their diet plans even after reducing their weight. In this way, they can ensure a healthy weight forever.

Fast Periodically

> "The best of all medicines is resting and fasting."
> Benjamin Franklin

Fasting is about not eating food voluntarily for varying lengths of time to keep your body and mind healthy. It is used as a therapy and observed by many religions across the world, including Islam, Hinduism, Buddhism, Christianity, Judaism, and Jainism. Mahatma Gandhi fasted during India's freedom struggle. He used it as a weapon to fight against the British to achieve India's independence and ensure peace in the

Indian society.

There are several types of fasting, including intermittent fasting, partial fasting, water fasting, and juice fasting. In intermittent fasting, intake is completely or partially restricted for a few hours up to a few days at a time, and resuming intake on other days. In water fasting, there is an intake of only water for a set amount of time. In juice fasting, there is an intake of vegetable or fruit juice for a certain period. In partial fasting, the intake of certain foods is eliminated from the diet for a set period. In intermittent fasting, people decide when to eat and when to abstain from eating. It is also known as cyclic fasting and is widely practiced globally. It shields your body from serious Type 2 diabetes. Research shows that regular intermittent fasting results in insulin resistance being reduced by about 30% and fasting blood sugar by about 5%.

Advantages and Disadvantages of Fasting

"All the vitality and all the energy I have comes to me because my body has been purified by fasting." Gandhi

There are innumerable benefits of fasting. It keeps your body light, energizes your mind, burns your fat, and increases your willpower. It improves the immunity of body, treats heart disorders, checks overweight, overcomes depression and cancer, reprograms cells, and treats diseases of the digestive system. It improves insulin sensitivity, increases your metabolism, and improves your verbal memory. It balances your hormones and increases your ability to use fat stores in your body. It beats addictions, normalizes food cravings, clears the skin, and whitens the eyes. Precisely, fasting is the strongest weapon against disease and illness. It is an operation without any surgery. Studies show that fasting can increase levels of human growth hormone (HGH), an important protein hormone that plays a role in growth, metabolism, weight loss, and muscle strength. However, there are disadvantages involved in fasting. It leads to body odor, hunger pangs, bad breath, headache, and cramps. The American Cancer Society reports that there are many short-term side effects of fasting. These include headaches, dizziness, lightheadedness, fatigue, low blood pressure, and abnormal heart rhythms. Fasting is not advisable for pregnant women and those who breastfeed. It is always advisable to consult with your doctor before embarking on a fast.

When you eat less, you live longer and are happier. Hence, fast periodically to overall your body system, ensure great health, and lead your life meaningfully.

Conclusion

"Weight loss can change your whole character. That always amazed me: Shedding pounds does change your personality. It changes your philosophy of life because you recognize that you are capable of using your mind to change your body." Jean Nidetch

Fad diets don't serve people in the long run because they may lack essential nutrients and slow down metabolism. Above all, the supplements may be dangerous. When you want to have weight loss happen realistically, it is advisable to avoid fad diets and welcome a healthy lifestyle. To conclude, improve your physical fitness by doing aerobic exercises such as swimming and water aerobics, resistance training, flexibility training, and lifestyle modification.

"After a lifetime of losing and gaining weight, I get it. No matter how you slice it, weight loss comes down to the simple formula of calories in, calories out." Valerie Bertinelli

References
http://time.com/5547500/exercise-live-longer
http://time.com/collection/guide-to-weight-loss
https://eatrunlift.me/eat-run-lift/2018/2/25/advantages-and-disadvantages-of-intermittent-fasting
https://healthyeating.sfgate.com/disadvantages-fasting-5546.html
https://www.healthline.com/nutrition/11-ways-to-increase-hgh#section7
https://www.businessinsider.in/How-to-look-and-feel-healthier-in-one-month-according-to-science/Stay-hydrated-with-plenty-of-water-and-maybe-even-some-coffee-if-thats-your-thing-/slideshow/64670076.cms
https://www.businessinsider.in/How-to-look-and-feel-

healthier-in-one-month-according-to-science/Stay-hydrated-with-plenty-of-water-and-maybe-even-some-coffee-if-thats-your-thing-/slideshow/64670076.cms

19 – Stay Younger and Live Longer

"If you live to be one hundred, you've got it made. Very few people die past that age." George Burns

Some people are scared of their old age. Most of them want to stay young forever. It is the law of nature to age. However, we can remain youthful to some extent with some foods, practices, habits, and hobbies and age gracefully. In this concluding chapter, we will discuss staying younger and living longer.

Facts and Findings on Aging

"The body is a sacred garment. It's your first and last garment; it is what you enter life in and what you depart life with, and it should be treated with honor." Martha Graham

Research shows that the majority of people over the age of 65 have Alzheimer's disease. Additionally, people with mild cognitive impairment (MCI) develop Alzheimer's disease. Age and family history are responsible for Alzheimer's disease. Here are some facts and findings on aging. Personality changes with age. Memory loss is a normal part of aging. Depression occurs more frequently in older adults than in younger adults. Older people perspire less, so they are more likely to suffer from hyperthermia. Osteoporosis is a normal part of the aging process for women. Most older adults lose interest in and capacity for sexual relations. All five senses tend to decline with advancing age. Older people are increasingly targets for fraud and scams. Retirement is often detrimental to health—i.e., people seem to become ill or die soon after retirement. Older adults are less anxious about death than are younger adults. Most older people are living in nursing homes. The modern family no longer takes care of its elderly. Hence, there is an urgent need for social security measures for older adults. Most older adults become set in their ways and are resistant to change. Older people tend to become more religious as they grow older. Older people do not adapt as well as younger age groups when they relocate to a new environment. Older adults take longer to recover from physical and psychological stress. Older females exhibit better healthcare practices than older males.

Tips to Stay Younger and Live Longer

"Those who regularly interact with their friends and peers are often the happiest and the healthiest, especially when social connections are maintained and preserved throughout a lifetime." Alexis Abramson Ph.D. Gerontologist

Research conducted by Dr. Dean Ornish and his team at the University of California, San Francisco concluded that following a program of "healthy eating, exercise, and stress reduction can not only reverse some diseases—it may slow down the aging process at the genetic level." Ikaria2 is the island where people forget to die. The Ikarians lead a simple lifestyle. The Ikarian diet is unique and features fresh vegetables, fruits, herbs, spices, and local honey, which are all products of weekly harvests that every citizen contributes to and benefits from, thereby maintaining a social structure that nurtures the entire community. Dan Buettner, Author of Blue Zones, remarked, "If you pay careful attention to the way Ikarians have lived their lives, it appears that a dozen subtly powerful, mutually enhancing, and pervasive factors are at work."

The factors that contribute to longevity include heredity, environment, and lifestyle. Hence, bring changes in the environment and your lifestyle. Here are some tips to stay younger and live longer. Start at an early age of life with good practices and habits to age gracefully. Acquire resilience. Build a strong social network. Eat a nutritious diet, with plenty of fruits and vegetables. Eat uncooked garlic. Avoid overeating. Stop eating when you feel only about 90 percent full. Drink an adequate quantity of water daily.

Exercise regularly. Do a workout in the water. Have sex regularly. Take a nap regularly. Live in the present instead of worrying about your unpleasant past and unpredictable future. Don't be idle. Keep yourself busy in pursuing your passionate hobbies. Keep your mind calm and quiet. Read good books. Wear clothes that the youth wear. Wear sunglasses and a hat. Wear safety glasses or goggles. Avoid smoking. Surround yourself with healthy people with positive vibes. Love your neighborhood. Socialize with others. Avoid loneliness as it increases blood pressure and raises the risk of death from stroke and heart disease. Develop an attitude of gratitude. Treat your life as a gift from God.

In my personal life, I look extremely youthful for my age. I enjoy interacting with young people to remain energetic and enthusiastic. When I served in educational institutions, students approached and interacted with me regularly. Currently, I go to the gym every day and interact with young people to inspire them with my ideas and insights.

Age Gracefully

"Aging is an inescapable process—aging well is a conscious choice." Alexis Abramson, Ph.D. Gerontologist

Globally, longevity is rising with increased healthcare facilities. Although people will have lots of diseases they will live longer due to better healthcare facilities. The financial institutions, banks, and insurance companies have realized it and started to tap the market globally.

Currently, people care more about how well they live than how long they live. Hence, emphasizes leading a quality and healthy life rather than leading a long life with diseases and illness.

"Listen to the aged…
For they will tell you about living and dying.

For they will enlighten you about problem-solving, sexuality, grief, sensory deprivation, and survival.
For they will teach you how to be courageous, loving, and generous." Irene Burnside

"The paradox of our time in history is that we have taller buildings but shorter tempers, wider Freeways, but narrower viewpoints. We spend more, but have less; we buy more, but enjoy less. We have bigger houses and smaller families, more conveniences, but less time. We have more degrees but less sense, more knowledge, but less judgment, more experts, yet more problems, and more medicine, but less wellness. ... We have multiplied our possessions, but reduced our values. We talk too much, love too seldom, and hate too often. We've learned how to make a living, but not a life. We've added years to life but not life to years. We've been to the moon and back, but have trouble crossing the street to meet a new neighbor." Bob Moorehead

References

https://www.bmo.com/assets/pdfs/gam/BMO-Report-Living-to-100-en.pdf
www.lsuagcenter.com/nr/rdonlyres/5131510b.../agingmythsandfactspowerpoint.ppt
https://www.bmo.com/assets/pdfs/gam/BMO-Report-Living-to-100-en.pdf
www.uky.edu/~hadleyr/PA2009/Kelly.ppt

References

Author's Vision 2030:

https://professormsraovision2030.blogspot.com

Author's Amazon URL: http://www.amazon.com/M.-S.-Rao/e/B00MB63BKM

Author's LinkedIn:

https://in.linkedin.com/in/professormsrao

Author's YouTube:

http://www.youtube.com/user/profmsr7

Author's Meta page:

https://www.facebook.com/Professor-MS-Rao-451516514937414/

Author's Company Meta Page:

https://www.facebook.com/MSR-Leadership-Consultants-India-375224215917499/

Author's Instagram:

https://www.instagram.com/professormsrao

Author's Blogs:

http://professormsraoguru.blogspot.com

http://professormsrao.blogspot.com

http://profmsr.blogspot.com

https://www.amazon.com/gp/product/B07P64KDF3

https://timesofindia.indiatimes.com/life-style/health-fitness/de-stress/make-joy-your-gps/articleshow/68109225.cms
https://news.harvard.edu/gazette/story/2018/04/5-healthy-habits-may-increase-life-expectancy-by-decade-or-more/
https://www.afpafitness.com/
https://www.livestrong.com/article/133041-importance-sports-health/
https://www.betterhealth.vic.gov.au/health/healthyliving/food-and-your-life-stages
https://www.entrepreneur.com/article/226179
https://www.alzheimers.net/foods-that-induce-memory-loss/
https://www.eatthis.com/healthy-foods-that-increase-sexual-stamina/
https://www.medicinenet.com/aerobic_exercise/article.htm#what_is_aerobic_exercise
https://www.mirror.co.uk/lifestyle/health/having-positive-mental-attitude-key-12714940
https://www.prevuemeetings.com/spark-blog/flip-the-script/integrate-wellness-meeting-like-pro/
https://www.hsidn.org/uploads/6/6/8/7/66873073/water_powerpoint.pptx
http://www.klientsolutech.com/importance-of-water/

https://www.nimh.nih.gov/health/publications/attention-deficit-hyperactivity-disorder-adhd-the-basics/index.shtml
https://kidshealth.org/en/parents/adhd.html
https://www.additudemag.com/what-is-adhd-symptoms-causes-treatments/
https://www.additudemag.com/adhd-diet-nutrition-sugar/
https://thetruthaboutcancer.com/signs-you-need-to-detox/
http://uk.complex.com/style/2015/04/how-to-dress-for-your-body-type-men/dressing-for-tall-men-dressing-for-short-men
http://upstatecouture.com/beauty/10-beauty-tips-how-to-look-more-attractive-in-one-month/
https://fashionista.com/2017/03/model-fashion-problems-treatment-abuse-health
https://www.lifehack.org/articles/lifestyle/8-important-lessons-stoic-philosophy-will-teach-you-about-being-happy.html
https://dailystoic.com/anthony-long/
https://classicalwisdom.com/philosophy/actionable-philosophy/
https://dailystoic.com/category/interviews/
http://time.com/5547500/exercise-live-longer
http://time.com/collection/guide-to-weight-loss
https://eatrunlift.me/eat-run-lift/2018/2/25/advantages-and-disadvantages-of-intermittent-fasting

https://healthyeating.sfgate.com/disadvantages-fasting-5546.html
https://www.healthline.com/nutrition/11-ways-to-increase-hgh#section7
https://www.businessinsider.in/How-to-look-and-feel-healthier-in-one-month-according-to-science/Stay-hydrated-with-plenty-of-water-and-maybe-even-some-coffee-if-thats-your-thing-/slideshow/64670076.cms
https://www.bmo.com/assets/pdfs/gam/BMO-Report-Living-to-100-en.pdf
www.lsuagcenter.com/nr/rdonlyres/5131510b.../agingmythsandfactspowerpoint.ppt
https://www.bmo.com/assets/pdfs/gam/BMO-Report-Living-to-100-en.pdf
www.uky.edu/~hadleyr/PA2009/Kelly.ppt
http://www.who.int/news-room/fact-sheets/detail/depression
https://www.medicalnewstoday.com/kc/depression-causes-symptoms-treatments-8933
https://www.psychologytoday.com/intl/blog/just-listen/201704/breaking-through-suicidal-mind
https://www.ncbi.nlm.nih.gov/pmc/articles/PMC533861/
https://psychcentral.com/blog/6-steps-for-beating-depression/
www.health.harvard.edu

Epilogue

"If you want happiness for an hour, take a nap. If you want happiness for a day, go fishing. If you want happiness for a year, inherit a fortune. If you want happiness for a lifetime, help someone else." Chinese proverb

We have authored this book to emphasize health and wealth to lead your life with purpose and meaning. If this book helps you excel as a health-conscious individual, it will have done its job. If you put this book down feeling that you are better equipped to lead a healthy lifestyle, we feel that our work as authors has been accomplished.

We would sincerely appreciate your invaluable feedback to facilitate improvements to this book. You may reach out to us via email: profmsr14@gmail.com.

We conduct presentations and workshops focusing on learning and leadership. Please do not hesitate to contact us should you require our services to assist in achieving your individual and organizational objectives. We find great fulfillment in offering consultation on wellness, leadership mentoring, and executive coaching. Additionally, we encourage you to follow our blogs:

http://professormsraovision2030.blogspot.com,
http://profmsr.blogspot.com,

http://professormsrao.blogspot.com, and http://professormsraoguru.blogspot.com.

These blogs pertain to learning, leadership, coaching, executive education, and mindfulness. If you find them interesting, please share the links with your friends, as knowledge grows when shared.

You may share your thoughts about *Self-Care: Stay Younger and Live Longer* on social media channels including Meta, X, and LinkedIn. We would appreciate a review on your blogs, websites, Amazon, or other online bookseller sites.

We genuinely hope that you found our book enjoyable and that it proved to be a useful, practical, and applicable resource. Should you wish to provide copies to your friends, colleagues, or employees, we are pleased to offer bulk discounts, which can include a personalized note and our signature.

Thank you for reading *Self-Care: Stay Younger and Live Longer*. We wish you great happiness and success, both in your business and in your life.

Sincerely,

Professor M.S. Rao, Ph.D
M. Padmavathy

List of Books Published by the Author

- See the Light in You: Acquire Spiritual Powers to Achieve Mindfulness, Wellness, Happiness, and Success

- Strategies to Build Women Leaders Globally: Think Managers, Think Men; Think Leaders, Think Women

- 21 Success Sutras for CEOs: How Global CEOs Overcome Leadership Challenges in Turbulent Times to Build Good to Great Organizations

- Secrets of Successful Public Speaking: How to Become a Great Speaker

- 21 Success Sutras for Leaders

- Spark: The Power to Become Big is Within You!

- Success Tools for CEO Coaches: Be a Learner, Leader and Ladder

- Smart Leadership: Lessons for Leaders

- Soft Leadership: A New Direction to Leadership

- Soft Leadership: Make Others Feel More Important

- Soft Leadership: An Innovative Leadership Style to Resolve Conflicts Amicably through Soft Skills and Negotiation Skills to Achieve Global Stability,

Peace, and Prosperity

- Soft Leadership: Acquire Leadership Ideas and Insights on Visionary, Inspirational, and Life Leadership to Stand Out as a Soft Leader Globally
- Soft Skills: Your Step-by-Step Guide to Overcome Workplace Challenges to Excel as a Leader
- Soft Skills for Students: Classroom to Corporate
- Soft Skills: Enhancing Employability
- Spirit of Indian Youth: Soft Skills for Young Managers
- Shortlist Your Employer: Acquire Soft Skills to Achieve Your Career and Leadership Success to Excel as a CEO
- Soft Skills: Toward A Sanctimonious Discipline Globally
- Success Can Be Yours
- Stand Out! Build a Successful Career and Become a Global Leader
- Secrets of Your Leadership Success: The 11 Indispensable E's of a Leader
- Sharpen Your Mind: Acquire Tools to Achieve Your Success

- Strategies for Improving Your Business Communication: The Book for Leaders to Communicate and Achieve Professional Success
- Smartness Guide: Success Tools for Students
- Sage Advice for Students and Educators: Stay Inspired!
- Soup for Academic Leaders: Acquire Teaching Tools to Achieve Your Academic Leadership Success
- Spot Your Leadership Style: Build Your Leadership Brand
- Secrets for Success: Failure is only a Comma, Not a Full Stop
- Soar Like Eagles! Success Tools for Freshers
- Student Leaders: Growing From Students To CEOs
- Success Sutras for Students: Stay Inspired!
- Striking Stories on Love and Romance: Spread the Message of Love
- Students: Concerns and Clarifications on Career, Entrepreneurship and Leadership Success
- Sutras for CEOs: Acquire Leadership Wisdom from Global Leadership Gurus

- Stay Hungry: Leadership Lessons from Leadership Gurus for Leaders and CEOs
- Sutras from Management Gurus: Sage Advice for Learners, Leaders and CEOs
- Stand Out as a Global Leader: Strive for Global Peace and Prosperity to Make a Difference
- Success Guide: An Inspirational Guide to Excel as a Leader and CEO
- Sharing Knowledge on Career, Leadership and Success: Improve Your Attitude and Personality to Excel as a Leader
- Short Stories on Life Leadership: Life is Beautiful!
- Professor M.S. Rao's Vision 2030: One Million Global Leaders
- Sharing Leadership Ideas and Insights: Moments and Memories on Indian Educational Institutions through Storytelling
- Start Leading: Acquire Leadership Lessons from Coaching, Mentoring and Leadership Experts
- School Leadership: Faculty First, Students Second, And Institutions Third
- Sharing in Success! A Guide to Acquire Insights on

Academic, Career, Leadership and Entrepreneurial Success

- Success Principles from Management Thinkers: Acquire Leadership Lessons to Create Winning Organization
- Simplify Your Leadership Strategies: How Great Leaders Build Successful Organizations That Win
- Stop Talking and Start Leading
- Success Principles to Thought Leadership: Learn Leadership Lessons from International Management Thinkers
- COVID-19: Humans' Search for Humanity
- Spiritual Tourism: A Guide to Your Enlightenment and Entertainment
- Spiritual Leadership: Stop Existing and Start Living
- Strategy: Leadership Lessons from Historical Leaders
- Secrets to Achieve Your Entrepreneurial and Leadership Success
- Self-Care: Stay Younger and Live Longer

Making a Positive Difference in the World

If you have been inspired by *Self-Care: Stay Younger and Live Longer* and want to help others lead their lives with purpose and meaning, and help Professor M. S. Rao, here are some ways you can do that:

- Gift *Self-Care* to your friends, family, and colleagues at work.

- Share your thoughts about *Stay Self-Care* on X, Meta, and blogs, or write a book review.

- Create a group to work through *Self-Care* together, sharing ideas and insights with others.

- If you are responsible for developing people within your organization, you can invest in copies of this book for all your leaders, managers, and teams.

About The Book

"He who is of a calm and happy nature will hardly feel the pressure of age, but to him who is of an opposite disposition, youth and age are equally a burden." Plato

This book shares the authors' years of experience in health, fitness, food, nutrition, cooking, modeling, and beauty. It explores self-care and explains leading a healthy lifestyle. It defines the perfect day and implores us to build character to become a champion. It explains attitude, encourages participation in physical activities and events, and advises making fitness an integral part of life. It emphasizes eating a variety of foods to stay healthy. It lists the foods to eat to boost your memory power. It outlines tips to improve your image and offers techniques to become a successful model. It calls you to eat to live, not live to eat. It outlines tips, tools, and techniques to stay younger and live longer. It elaborates on the causes, effects, and remedies for depression. It offers tools and techniques to prevent suicidal thoughts to build a blissful, peaceful, and prosperous world.

This is a book on life leadership outlining health, food, nutrition, fitness, modeling, and beauty, and is written from a practitioner's perspective. You can easily toss the book into a briefcase or purse and read here and there as time allows. It is a quick reference guide for all learners, leaders, and entrepreneurs.

About The Authors

Professor M.S. Rao, Ph.D.
The Father of Soft Leadership
Vision 2030:

http://professormsraovision2030.blogspot.com

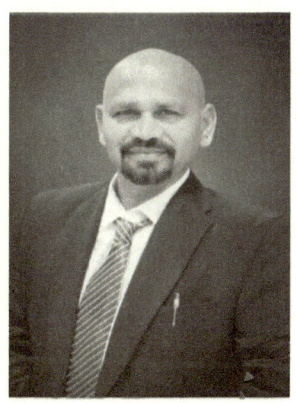

Professor M.S. Rao, Ph.D., is a 21st-Century Philosopher & the Father of "Soft Leadership." He is an International Leadership Guru and the Founder of MSR Leadership Consultants, India. He has forty-four years of diversified experience, including military, and is the author of fifty-five books, including the bestselling *'See the Light in You'* URL:https://www.amazon.com/See-Light-You-Spiritual-Mindfulness/dp/1949003132.

He is a columnist and an author-at-large at Entrepreneur. He has published over 300 papers and articles in prestigious international publications, including *Leader to Leader, Thunderbird International Business Review, Strategic HR Review, Development and Learning in Organizations, Industrial and Commercial Training, On the Horizon,* and *Entrepreneur magazine.* He is a soldier, entrepreneur, editor, educator, author, explorer, enlightener, thinker, writer, researcher, mentor, motivator, professor, reformer, traveler, blogger, storyteller, volunteer, activist, futurist, analyst, strategist, and coach. He is a C-Suite advisor and global keynote speaker. He brings a strategic eye and long-range vision, given his multifaceted professional experience including military, teaching, training, research, consultancy, and philosophy. He is passionate about serving and making a difference in the lives of others. He trains a new generation of leaders through leadership education and publications.

He hopes to build one million students as global leaders by 2030.

URL: http://professormsraovision2030.blogspot.com/2014/12/professor-m-s-raos-vision-2030-one_31.html.

He volunteers for peace activities, advocates gender equality (#HeForShe), and builds students globally. He invests his time in authoring books and blogging on executive education, learning, and leadership. Most of his work is free of charge on his four blogs, including http://professormsraovision2030.blogspot.com.

He is a prolific author and a dynamic, energetic, and inspirational leadership speaker. He can be reached at profmsr14@gmail.com.

M. Padmavathy is an award-winning author, image consultant, expert chef, and beautician. She can be reached at mpadmavathy14@gmail.com.